MW01233322

K. Boytek is an American author born and raised in West Virginia. Her first book, *Growing Spiritually with Schedules, Spouses, Toddlers, and Pre-Teens: An Unfiltered Guide for the Busy Mom Life*, is based on her experience as a mother, as a former child victim advocate and from extensive self-education in mind, body, and spirit along with conscious parenting teachings. Her book is centered around spiritual awareness and mindful parenting. It serves as a self-growth guide on becoming a better person and parent.

"Growth is ever-flowing on the spiritual journey. It's never too late for anything."

– K. Boytek

My mom and dad, I'd like to thank you for being such amazing parents. I cannot thank you both enough for all you have done for me, all you have taught me, and all you continue to do and teach. You are my mentors and my best friends. Thank you.

My grandparents and sister, thank you for the unconditional love and support you have always given me. You bring so much happiness to my life and all those who know you. I love you all so very much.

My children, my two beautiful girls, you have completed my life and filled my heart with pure love. I started this journey with you both as my focus. You both have been and will always be my purpose. I love you both to the moon and back. Forever.

The higher, infinite source from which this book derived, I humbly thank you for your enlightenment, for your guidance, and for your peace.

K. Boytek

GROWING SPIRITUALLY WITH SCHEDULES, SPOUSES, TODDLERS, AND PRE-TEENS

AN UNFILTERED GUIDE FOR THE BUSY MOM LIFE

AUSTIN MACAULEY PUBLISHERS™

LONDON • CAMBRIDGE • NEW YORK • SHARJAH

Copyright © K. Boytek (2021)

Ordering Information
Quantity sales: Special discounts are available on quantity purchases by corporations, associations, and others. For details, contact the publisher at the address below.

Publisher's Cataloging-in-Publication data
Boytek, K.
Growing Spiritually with Schedules, Spouses, Toddlers, and Pre-Teens

ISBN 9781643787114 (Paperback)
ISBN 9781643787893 (Hardback)
ISBN 9781645361688 (ePub e-book)

Library of Congress Control Number: 2021901431

www.austinmacauley.com/us

First Published (2021)
Austin Macauley Publishers LLC
40 Wall Street, 33rd Floor, Suite 3302
New York, NY 10005
USA

mail-usa@austinmacauley.com
+1 (646) 5125767

Thank you for sparing time to grow with me. I hope this book helps you, like it helped me, on your journey to a more fulfilled life! Happy reading!

– K. Boytek

Author's Note

You may have noticed this book isn't a 'short' book. You may have thought, why does she think this is a quick read or a quick guide for the busy life, for the busy mom? This book isn't something you're going to finish in a day, never promised that, but it is something you can read throughout your day and on all your quick breaks from everyday hustle and bustle. I have jam packed this book with quick tips and helpful guidelines that will help you grow on your spiritual journey, all the while not requiring hours of your time to study. I'm dropping mom bombs, ya'll (spiritually speaking).

This book is laid out so that you can sit in the car line waiting to get your kids and learn a little something new within those, however few minutes. It's something you can read on potty break without feeling like you read a bunch of words that didn't reach the point in the amount of time you had available. So now you're going to have to go back and re-read all of it so that you can grasp the concept it was trying to teach you.

If one of the processes I have in this book takes a bit of time, I'll let you know beforehand, so that you can scroll on for something that won't require as much time, if you happen to be limited. If you know you only have five minutes to spare, skip to the tips, you can read the rest later. I wanted to make sure if all you had was 30 seconds today, that I had put something in this book you could grab onto quickly to apply immediately. So, if you're struggling with balancing it all, don't feel bad if you don't get a chapter read, you can come back later. This was written with your busy schedule in mind.

Table of Contents

Invitation

Have you ever watched a television show, heard a story, or maybe you saw a magazine article in the grocery store checkout lane of someone, somewhere that made their life better by practicing spiritual awareness? Surely, you have heard of this spiritual movement that so many are learning and applying to their lives, one by one, stating facts of the life changes and miracles they've received all by putting action behind this powerful knowledge. I'm sure you, like me, saw this and thought to yourself, WOW! That's awesome. I want to learn that. How can I do that?

An immediate rush of excitement and anticipation floods your system as you think of the possibilities this could bring to your life. Then, without warning a high-pitched scream startles you out of your daydream and your two-year-old, without saying a word, reminds you that you do not have extra time in your day to shower without an audience, let alone spend hours studying these life-changing skills that may or may not work.

Well, my fellow mothers, I invite you to take a small break of your world filled with cleaning, cooking, dirty diapers, after school ball games, birthday parties, laundry pile ups and the never-ending life of motherhood to grow with me on this amazing journey that's going to change your life for the better. Even if you can only read a few pages while child number one is in school and child number two is napping, I promise you it will be worth it! So, put down those crayons you're picking up and don't even think about touching that Facebook app and let's begin.

Chapter One
Definition

Spiritual Awareness or Spiritual Awakening is the process by which we begin to explore our own being in order to become whole and reunite our spirit with our physical bodies in a commonality of purpose.

OK. GREAT. Now we have the 'google' definition, but let's break it down even further. What exactly does that mean? Do I feel (not) whole? I already know who I am, right? I feel like I do, I feel like I know everything there is to know about me. I mean, I have known me my whole life. These are the questions I asked myself when I began my journey. I remember one thought that kept reappearing in my brain. I don't need to know who I am, I already know that, I just want to know how to achieve my dreams and goals while being the best mom I can be, passing what I know down to my children.

Let's take this as a jumping off point. Most of us reading this book, I'm assuming because of my suggestive title, are mothers. Moms. Working moms, stay at home moms, stepmoms, grandmothers, great grandmothers, what do we all have in common ladies? … KIDS. We all have or have had at some point tiny little humans looking to us for their every need. Literally every need, from feeding and wiping butts, to broken hearts that need soothed and college degrees. We have been the person, their person, that has had to lay the path, teach the wrongs and rights and hope with our entire being that the things we were and are teaching stick and help them be the best they can be in this life. It's scary, there isn't a manual for us to look in when our nine-year-old daughter asks why boys can pee standing up! I mean come on, how easy would that be to say, "Hang on, sweetie, while I get my 'how to mom the right way book' for an answer." No, instead our faces show our emotions and we scrabble trying to find the perfect age-appropriate answer. Bottom line, MOMMING IS HARD.

Now add spirituality into the mix, with so many different beliefs out there how do I find the one for me? How do I point my kids to the right one? How do I even know it's the right one? I'm so pleased to tell you the answer is SIMPLE (I know, not a word you're that familiar with); nevertheless, it is so simple. IT FEELS GOOD. Not buying a new pair of shoes good. This GOOD is absolute and pure, it settles with your soul, you don't second-guess, it just is. This good is true and you have zero doubt in any of it.

I remember my first encounter with learning a spiritual truth. I was with my mom, I was younger, late teens, early 20s and I felt lost. I wasn't sure where to go with my life or if I was making the best decisions for myself. So I went to my mom. I remember asking her, "How do I know? What's something I can look to and ask when I'm thinking of or about to make a decision? I need guidance." My mother's reply to me is something I still use in my everyday choices, she said, "If it feels good without any unsettling feelings or bad thoughts attached and if it brings only happiness and goodness to you and those in your life, then it is of the spirit and you can rest assured that you will be fine with that choice. However, if it feels bad, leaves any empty feelings or will bring pain, suffering or hurt to you or anyone in your life now or later on, then that is not the best decision, not of the spirit and you need to walk away from it."

You would think knowing right and wrong would come into play here, but for me it was fuzzy. As an adult it's not always black and white, so right and wrong just wasn't working. It wasn't enough, I needed a more 'adult answer' of something that could help me with my life choices. When we grow up, we tend to lose some of the platforms we based our decisions on when we were seven. It's no longer do I want to play barbies or jump on the trampoline, it's grown-up stuff with grown up consequences. Every cause has an effect. Every decision will result in a different tomorrow. The knowledge you have and apply today is what affects the later outcome. That applies to everything in your life, including the decisions you make with your children. What you tell them today will affect their tomorrow. Your children will see the choices you make and more than likely, at some point, make similar choices. That is why becoming spiritually enlightened/spiritually awakened is so important. It will clarify the path you take in every aspect of your life. This not only will help you, but also helps them.

Once this small truth is practiced you will notice how much better your mind feels when it comes to making decisions. The stress will be off of your shoulders as you simply replace the worry and anxiety with the small question. Will this bring only good or will this possibly bring something bad. You will have a clear answer every time. If both choices feel good, then just pick one! You have two great choices. If they both feel bad or have some long-term yucky feeling, walk away, something better will come along, don't settle for something just because it was the lesser of the two 'yucky' feelings. The act of practicing this will help you in re-creating yourself.

Remember earlier when I said I thought I knew who I was, the answer is yes. I did know who my ego driven worldly self was. Was she bad? Not necessarily. Was she fully empowered by her spiritual self? No.

So, then this opens a door. Do I stay where I am, having some good days, some great days, some okay days and some bad days? Always looking for ways to better my life, my kids' life, my family and our future, but leaving it at that. Always looking. Or do I shed my self-image, shed the person I and everyone that has ever known me 'knows' to embrace this enlightened source of spiritual understanding, this secret knowledge that will manifest all my desires for the greater good. I'll leave that up to you to decide, just remember to practice that little skill I mentioned.

I'll see you in the next chapter.

Ps. It's All a Scam?

It's been said that positive thinking, practicing the law of attraction, and studying this type of releasing self-doubt spiritual awakening is a pyramid scheme, a scam. Just like with anything else, you're going to run into people that, have a better way, tried it but never saw results, think it's just another self-help book of BS or people that simply don't believe in it.

I'm not writing this book to argue. I'm not trying to convince you of anything. I'm saying, listen up! This really worked for me. I'm busy, I don't have time to take classes or go on a peace retreat, I need something that I can literally read while I'm using the potty. I have kids, two kids! I want a better life yes, of course, but I also must do my part in keeping what I have right now together and as happy as possible, so my 'learning time' is limited. I have tried everything I am willing to try, by that I mean, it's not my personal choice to try snake handling for spiritual awakening. I don't personally feel my spirit leading me in that direction and I can only go where I feel my inner pull take me. I'm following my inside source of knowledge, my gut, I'm following what is being presented to me from the higher power.

I'm not trying to tell you or anyone else that my source is smarter than your source because this is the path I've taken. I believe it's the same source in us all; it's a higher consciousness, a brighter path, an enlightened future. While this may sound fairy tale La La Land to some, or totally bonkers to others, that's fine. Stop reading. Choose to put this book down. Your opinion of me is none of my business. I'm writing this to share my personal experience and knowledge I have gained and benefitted from with you, in hopes that it helps you achieve a happier life and helps you in becoming the best person you can be. That's it. If it's not for you then I still wish you the same thing, happiness in your life. If it is for you, great! Practice these tips and apply them to your life, see if they work for you like they did for me and let's keep going!

Chapter Two
Forgiveness of Self

Spirit:

The nonphysical part of a person which is the seat of emotions and character; the soul.

REPEAT. REPEAT. REPEAT.

Nonphysical part also known as: THE GUT, THE INTUITION.

Emotions also known as: THE FEELS, THE ROLLER COASTER of HAPPY and SAD.

Character also known as: MORAL QUALITIES, YOUR PERSONALITY.

I'd like to take a moment to make a statement. I do not have any intention on you changing your wonderful qualities, why would I? If they are wonderful then they are already in alignment with the spirit, my only intention is to help you become aware and awakened of the off-balance parts of you and your life for the purpose of simply enlightening you. What helps you helps your children and eventually all mankind. My purpose is to provide tips and skill sets that I have personally used to help make these changes in myself. I do not push anything that I haven't tried, tested and received the result. I have tried, I have tested, and I have graciously received the results of the things I'm telling/teaching you; I only wish for you to apply them to better your life. With that I salute you and I humbly thank you for making the decision to say, "It's time I make a change. I want a change. I want better and I deserve better."

Let's start with the nonphysical part which I am going to refer to hence forth as, THE GUT.

Have you ever felt it? That tiny little nudge that feels deep in your belly if something is off or extremely on. How often do you push it aside as worry or just your imagination running away with you? How often do you stop and listen? If you are one of those people that stop and listen, then how often do you lean the way its lead you to go? If you listen and apply this little nudge to your life, then insert applause here. If not, read on…

This is important! This is a built-in mechanism from the higher source, this is to help you. It's not meant to be pesky; it is meant to be helpful. If you have trouble telling the difference between what your head may be saying and what your gut is feeling, put the first tip into action (Chapter One: good or bad decision skill) and know that your gut will never lead you into anything that may bring harm or hurt into your life. It will only bring the best possible answer or solution before you. This step is short, sweet, and easy. Listen to your gut, follow your gut, and trust your gut. Put this tip into action.

Next, let's talk about emotions…The Feels…Oh, the feels, as a mother of two I can say that I know pretty much every emotion there is. I can tell if its surface emotion that just needs a booboo kiss or deep emotion that requires immediate attention followed up with a dose of Gilmore Girls Binge watching and popcorn. I've seen crocodile tears that suddenly stop as they catch a glimpse of their reflection in a mirror and tears from laughing so hard that you're literally crying. That's not all, I am also lucky enough to hear my two-year-old laugh in her pure and innocent way, just the most adorable giggles and I can share laughter with my sweet nine-year-old, who almost always has a bright, beautiful smile on her face. Emotions can feel wonderful or miserable, so here's the tip: Choose.

That's right! It's a choice again. I know you're thinking, okay I'm done with this book, you can't choose how something makes you feel, she's cray-cray, but hear me out. Studies show that it's physically impossible to monitor all your thoughts; there are too many. However, these thoughts provoke emotions, which you can control. YOU CAN CONTROL YOUR EMOTIONS. In return this helps you control your thought process.

How do you do this? Again, it's simple. If it feels good when you think about it, then think away! It's good to keep uplifting thoughts around that raise your spirits! Positive thinking should be at the top of your 'goals' list. If it feels bad when you think about it, then try this skill: Visualize this thought passing by in front of you, observe it, do not grab onto this thought and attach your emotions, just let it pass. If you make a habit of grabbing negative thoughts and becoming caught up in them, then that's exactly what you'll attract. More negative thoughts with negatively attached emotions. This is something that requires practice, it's not often you meet someone that says, "I never feel sad or bad." Most of the planet has just as many sad, bad or 'just okay' days, then on top of the world days, if you start asking around. That shouldn't be. Life is exciting, amazing and full of happiness. It's up to you what you choose to pick out of your story and focus on. If you think of something that upsets you, don't beat yourself up about it, just close your eyes and visualize placing the thought on a screen in front of you then let it pass by. Repeat this process every time you start to feel down or depressed or have negative thoughts. Replace this thought with a happy thought or think of something you're grateful for even if it's something as simple as running water. Feel that happy and grateful emotion within, let it sink into your core and shine out of you like a thousand shinning specs. Literally visualize your skin shinning with beautiful 'fairy dust' all the while producing this happy and completely selfless emotion. Doing this will retrain your brain to be in a more positive state.

Not every negative emotion can be dealt with in that way though, that's a tip intended for more of your 'laying on top' problems. Some things are more of an issue than waking up with your power off, hair not washed, kids have school in a half hour, and you feel like you opened your eyes to the collusion course on survivor island.

If your emotion is coming from a deep-rooted issue, maybe it's something you've carried with you since childhood or maybe it's a regret, multiple regrets or different things that have happened over periods of time; buildups. I'd like to tell you about my personal experience that has a skill for you to try. This skill helped me overcome my deep-rooted issues and attached emotions I had.

When I started writing this book, I made myself a promise that no matter how unfiltered or raw my tools I used to overcome were, I would describe them as accurately as possible, so here goes...

I carried a lot of regret and guilt with me that lasted around a five-to-seven-year span. This guilt and regret were extremely deep rooted, and it felt as though I was being haunted by my past. I felt like I truly could not escape the decisions I once made, like no one would truly forgive me and I would never truly forgive myself. I carried this with me into my spiritual journey; in fact, it wasn't until recently that I overcame this giant block in my soul. I mean that, it felt as if it were eating away at my very soul. I didn't know what to do. I had hit a wall with this emotion. I felt like I had tried all the tools I had learned and that they weren't working. Every time it surfaced, I felt as though I had made no progress. This in turn made me feel frustrated, sad, aggravated and hurt. Deep Hurt: To the Core Pain. How could I forgive this? I had done this, and I couldn't take it back. How could I let go of people's perception of who I was then? How could I recognize who I was and the things I had done as wrong, not of the spirit, not of higher consciousness, but forgive myself truly? I felt hate for the girl I used to be. How do you forgive someone you hate? This is what I did, descriptively...

Have you ever seen the movie Spiderman? There is a scene in the movie where the Spiderman character is being overtaken by this black, evil tar, this sticky substance that consumes him. I visualized that substance on me at the time I made those decisions. I visualized that substance consuming me from the inside out. I closed my eyes and saw me laying, in the fetal position, on the floor of my house I currently live in (I brought her, who I was then, visually, to my present self) with that evil tar all over her body, she/I was crying. I felt her pain, her aloneness, her extreme sadness, her guilt, her regret for all she had done to herself and the people she loved. I felt the judgment of everyone's opinions of her and how she had let them affect her self-image. I felt the desperation in her, wishing she could take it back. I FELT IT ALL.

Then, I visualized me, the NOW me. The more enlightened, growing spiritually everyday me, standing over her/me. I leaned down to her, laying my arms around her/my body and saying this:

I forgive you; I love you and I forgive you. You are loved.
ALL IS FORGIVEN AND YOU ARE LOVED.

I also sent all my emotion into her; I visually saw my emotion of love coming out of me and going into her body like a heat wave of energy, a heat wave of pure love. This love felt like the love I have for my children; the I'll never forsake you, I'll never abandon you, I'd give my life to save you and I will <u>always</u> have your back love. I attached my forgiveness and loving emotions together with my words and visually pushed them into her/me. I released any hate I had for the girl I was, emitting only love for this girl that was not on a spiritual path and didn't have the knowledge of an enlightened self at that time. A girl trapped by her own conditioning. I'm not saying what I did wasn't wrong; I'm simply forgiving the old me. I'm loving the spirit inside the girl I was that hadn't been allowed to shine yet.

This process of forgiveness of self (I have given it this name) was not easy. It was very emotional, and I waited to do it while my oldest child was in school and my toddler was down for her afternoon nap. It was messy with tears. I cried for a while after completing this visualization, but it wasn't a sad cry, it was a relief cry. A weight was lifting. Notice I said lifting and not lifted. I had to repeat this process three different times after that. Allowing my love for this girl I used to be to grow, allowing the energy wave I pushed into her to become stronger. After the fourth and final time, I knew I had accomplished true forgiveness of self. Myself. I had replaced my hate with love, pure love. There must be complete love, not love with holes poked in it and other emotions seeping in. This must be a solid love and forgiveness filled energy flow into the once broken you.

I don't know your journey, but I invite you to take this technique that truly worked for me and apply it for yourself. I may not have walked in your shoes, but I know that all of our spirits are like-minded. That's what makes this journey real. We are each other's counter points and when you're on this path you know what I'm saying to ring true. So, try it, forgive the old you so that you can embrace the beautiful new you.

Last, but not least…

Character. Your Personality.

At the beginning of this chapter, I made a statement that I thought I knew who I was. I later answered that statement by saying yes, I did know my ego driven worldly self. For the most part, whether you want to admit it or not, we as humans are driven by other people's opinions of us; what we have, what we wear, what we do, our own personal opinions of ourselves, how much money we have, the brands we buy, the car we drive and what the world perceives as acceptable, normal, high-quality, intelligent and important. We tend to let this develop our character. This may be difficult for you to accept because you may perceive this as an insult, it's not. That's the emotion you've CHOSEN to attach to it. So, let that emotion pass and just listen, open your mind. We were all born into a world that runs on time, runs on money, runs on social life and perception. Also, for us moms, runs on COFFEE. Which you will not hear me say one negative thing about, by the way, as I sip my 3rd cup. Why can I feel completely at ease with my coffee drinking obsession? Because it feels good. There is nothing bad attached, no negatives. I'm healthy and don't usually over drink so my love for this delicious beverage is fine. See how I applied the good or bad decision skill, Stress Be Gone!

Now back to what I was saying, that is the world we were born into and what's more, the world we learned all we know about everything in. I'm not saying you haven't learned great things. Taking a shower is great, dancing is great, showing your kids how to read is great! Even worldly things can be great: money, luxury, clothing. The list can go on and on. I know I may be starting to sound contradictory but bear with me. I'm not saying that these things aren't great. I'm not saying that everything in your personality needs changed or fixed. I'm saying that we need to put filter glasses on and learn to recognize what is truly of the spirit, truly good, things that will bring true happiness and things that won't.

Filter your world. This should provide the basis for any non-spiritual personality traits you're looking to replace. If you base your character on how many Facebook likes you have and you truly feel disheartened if your Instagram selfie only got one like, then I'm here to be your wakeup call, so to speak. That's not good. That thinking will always let you down at some point and you'll attach the emotion of sadness and self-pity to it, which is not of the spirit. My goal, your goal, OUR goal is to adapt our character to positive thoughts that in return bring about positive emotions. Why is this important? Because the happier you feel about who you are, the more you love yourself, not in a conceded way, but a pure 'I love me, my mind, body, spirit and soul way,' the more energy, which is vibration, you will produce in a positive outpour. Your outpour affects everything around you. It defines your character. Think about it, if you're having what you've perceived as a 'bad day' your outpour to your kids and spouse may be stern, you may sound hateful because of the stress you have packed around all day; this has a domino effect. Your kids will say either to you or under their breath as they walk away, mom's so hateful. Your spouse may say, I'm sorry you've had a bad day or if they've also allowed stress to affect their day, they may be hateful, playing your emotions right back to you, expressing tone and aggravation.

The law of attraction states that like attracts like. That couldn't be truer. Have you ever had an argument or thought about something someone did that made you upset and suddenly felt wonderful? No, you haven't. Why? Because of the emotion you have chosen to attach to this argument or this incident you've perceived to be upsetting. Your emotions and thoughts about this attracted the same thing back to you. Like attracts Like.

If you keep allowing things to pull you into negativity, then slowly the people around you will start to perceive things about your character because of your negative outpour. Your kids may say, "I love my mom and she's great, but sometimes she can be hateful if she's stressed." Not only are they adapting that to your personality, they are also viewing it as a normal thing for a hectic day or it's ok to have an attitude if your day hasn't gone how you thought it should. Your spouse may say, "I love my wife, but I could do without the nagging."

What did that statement just do? Under your traits it listed:

Loving
Kind
Happy
Hateful when stressed
Nagy

You chose to put emotions into play that changed your personality, making the people around you perceive you as something your true spirit, your true self, has no play in. Choose a different thought pattern. Choose a different emotion. No matter how frustrating you may be choosing to feel over whatever happened in your day, choose to change the course. Stop and think of something that made you feel amazing and shine that awesome outpour of vibration to everyone you meet, shine that outpour to your spouse, shine it to your children because that is your core personality. That is the personality of the spirit and that outpour will attract positive reactions and positive emotions right back to you. If you put out joy, you'll receive joy. If you put out kindness, you'll receive kindness. Make those qualities your character, make gratefulness for all you have and happiness for your life your personality.

TIP: A tip that will help in doing this is applying affirmation and autosuggestion. Say positive, uplifting things to yourself all day. Feel the emotion of gratitude, peace and joy for your life, be thankful for your wonderful existing personality traits and then be grateful for your new ones developing. Life is meant for you, specifically for you to be happy and fulfilled. Your spirit is already complete with peace, love, joy, strength, courage and faith, just let it rise within you.

YOU IS KIND, YOU IS SMART, YOU IS IMPORTANT.
-AIBILEEN CLARK, THE MOVIE 'THE HELP'

Chapter Three
Now Accepting Applications

I'd like for you to get a sheet of paper, if you can't find a blank sheet grab anything close by, the back of a target receipt or the back of one of your kid's school announcement papers will work just fine. Take a two-second break. Write down three things:

ASK
BELIEVE
RECEIVE

It's time to practice the law of attraction by submitting your first application.

But First: What is the law of attraction?

Law of Attraction is the belief that positive or negative thoughts bring positive or negative experiences into a person's life. The belief is based on the idea that people and their thoughts are both made from pure energy, and that through the process of like energy attracting like energy a person can improve their own health, wealth, and personal relationships. It is a Universal Law.

Throughout this chapter I will be focusing on the law of attraction and the three things you wrote: ASK. BELIEVE. RECEIVE.

First thing: ASK

Ask for what? ANYTHING. Does that seem too farfetched for you? No problem, that's completely fine, we are all starting at different levels where some things may seem like they're 'too much right now' and that's ok. The end goal will be the same with everyone. Let's start wherever you feel the most comfortable. Ask for something that seems obtainable to you, it can be whatever you wish it to be, IF you have complete, unwavering belief you will achieve the thing you ask for. I recently watched a show that I felt helped me tremendously with this practice (I will list this show, along with others, at the end of the book). A couple of examples I would suggest for you to ask for would be:

- A Beverage. Ask to receive a beverage from another source. It can be your favorite soda or a cup of tea, whatever you want, go wild! Just ask. Ask to receive it today, tomorrow, next Thursday, whenever you feel that what you're asking for is something you can put 100% of your faith (which is TRUST) in. Don't ask for something unrealistic, like not having to change a poop diaper this week, it must be something realistic that you feel completely comfortable with. With that being said, I stand by my statement that anything is obtainable. If you believe that in three months, you'll receive $50,000.00 dollars or complete health and you believe, want and desire that with zero doubt, with unwavering faith and complete trust, then that is what you'll receive. The key ingredient to the law of attraction is your desire must include a powerful emotion (which generates vibration) to back it up along with unwavering belief and trust that you can have it. If any of that is lacking, then you're simply left with wanting something badly. Since some of us are rookies at this practice, I feel that it's better to start smaller and work up from there, but if you're on a higher level currently then by all means, you ask for what you believe is truly obtainable by you.

- $5.00 Dollars. Ask that within a week you'll receive $5.00 extra dollars. Who do you ask? The universal energy that flows in and around you, the power that made you, the higher self-knowledge, ask the very thing you're searching for, higher consciousness, isn't that the reason you're still reading this book? Try it, ask. You must have full belief that you'll receive the thing you ask for. No doubt can be present. You asked for $5.00 extra dollars this week, now say to yourself. This week I WILL OBTAIN $5.00 EXTRA DOLLARS. NOT, I WANT TO OBTAIN $5.00 EXTRA DOLLARS. Afterward, thank the universal energy, the higher consciousness, for this gift. It's very important that you are truly grateful for the things that you're asking for and receive.

Some may feel that I am talking silly and some may think that you can't ask for things like that. You may even be thinking that to yourself as you're reading. If you have doubt in the higher power, the power that created you, the power that is the universal energy, that is complete enlightenment, then you will not succeed in this practice. Having doubt will poke holes in the belief system and your results will be mediocre at best. If you want something in this life, anything, and your subconscious thought process behind it is lack of eternal emotion for the thing you desire or self-doubt in your ability to achieve it. If, in the back of your mind, you always have a lingering thought of 'there's no way I can accomplish that' or 'that's too far of a stretch to think I could have that' then guess what, the universal energy says, "Your wish is my command," and you'll never receive it. You'll attract what you put out. Those statements are negative; you're doubting your abilities to receive something you truly desire, something you deserve. You're doubting that the infinite power can produce greater things for you.

Why? Why do you think you can't achieve all you want? Why would a powerful source create you, all of you, with all of your intricate detail, then give you all this energy, energy to heal, energy to keep up with your kids and schedule, put you in a world filled with so many beautiful material and non-materialistic things and then say to you, "Know your limits, don't soar to high, don't get carried away with yourself, conserve your energy, you can't have this, you can't have that. Live a mediocre life with a job you're not crazy about, grow old and then die." Do you think that type of negative energy applied to the power that created you? What if it didn't place within you the ability to heal a scratch. The power that made you is limitless. You derive from a limitless source. Start living with that knowledge. You are an amazing being that can achieve amazing things. Start living that way today!

TIP: When you are asking for these things you desire make sure to be clear, if you say, "Someday I'd like to have a decent car," you may not be happy 40 years from now when you're driving the car that was your next to last pick on the lot. Use clarity and be decisive in your choices, if you're foggy with your outpour, you'll receive a foggy result.

Second Thing: BELIEVE

This part is the most important part of the three-step process. You can say you believe in something, yet in the back of your mind you have doubts. It can be hard to shake those doubts. A lot of times they are a product of our past conditioning, things we've been taught our entire lives to not invest full trust in. Just remember, if you have doubts, you won't receive the full result. If your doubts are many and your emotion attached to them is strong, you may receive nothing. A lot of people that try and fail at practicing the law of attraction say that it doesn't work, that it's a scam. The only reason this practice wouldn't work for you or anyone else is because it's not being practiced correctly. Remind yourself that it takes time to retrain your thought process you have literally carried with you most of your life, especially your adult life. Don't be too hard on yourself, you're a student, this process is to make you feel better, be better and think better, nothing you learn should make you feel depressed or negative. There's no need in spending time being hard on yourself because of the progress you're making or not making. This isn't a race, those thoughts are hindering you on your journey. This is a negative thought process that brings about negative emotions and results in a negative outpour that will attract negative things to you and to your life. Lots of negatives. Shake that off. Choose to think another way and stop attaching to those emotions. You're once again falling into the routine of 'I'm not doing this right; I should be moving faster or why can't I see any physical changes.'

Did you find out you were pregnant and give birth to a healthy fully developed baby one week later? No, but why doesn't that make you feel like you weren't doing it right or like you should be developing your baby faster? Because you know that creating a human being takes time, it's a miracle. It's not an overnight achievement. You never get frustrated at the time it takes to have a full pregnancy because you know it is needed. This same statement could even be said about receiving a paycheck. You don't work Monday and Tuesday, then get upset if your paycheck isn't deposited after the two days of work you did. You know it takes time, usually every two weeks. Do you feel upset if you don't get your paycheck sooner? No.

Apply that understanding with this, stop expecting results as soon as you read a paragraph or definition in a book that's trying to help you achieve your desires and better your life. You must give the universal energy time to develop a plan and manifest your desires. You also may be required to put forth effort. You don't get abs without doing some sit-ups. Don't sit on your couch waiting for something to fall in your lap with no effort made. It may not always be a physical effort, but if it is, apply whatever is necessary. You will know what you need to do. If you have asked the universal energy, higher power, for something that's good. This also important, it cannot be a bad thing you ask for that could bring hurt or pain to you or those around you. And you invest you full confidence, trust, and belief that you WILL receive what you're wanting backed with strong desire (emotion) that makes your vibration powerful, you're going to get it. Not you might. You will! Just add the necessary ingredients. If I forget to add sugar to my peanut butter fudge, then I'll end up with a marshmallow cream and peanut butter swirl blob. If you forget to add unwavering belief in your recipe for a better life, you'll end up with exactly what you've attracted into it, your own personal, emotional, inconsistent living swirl blob.

Third Thing: RECEIVE

Here's the fun part! This is where your work of applying the knowledge you have learned pays off! Wahoo! Go You! I'm cheering you on. Congratulations!

Feel that? That feeling in your belly of overwhelming happiness, that smile on your face and light in your soul...that's the end goal. That's what we are working toward. Maybe you just signed the papers on your dream home, maybe you just drove off the car lot in your brand-new ride or maybe you healed your body of an ongoing health condition, whatever you manifested you have achieved by putting action behind your intentions to be better and allowing higher consciousness to be part of your everyday life. I want you to take that happiness you're feeling right now and add one ingredient. GRATEFULNESS. So, So, So Important. Be grateful for what the universal energy has given you, feel the gratefulness in the same way that you feel the joy. Let it flourish and shine out of you like an amazing golden light projecting from your very body. Visualize this light beaming from your physical body and now attach your positive emotion of joy and gratitude as you say aloud, "Thank you, Thank you, higher power/higher consciousness/universal energy."

TIP: Wake up every morning and say to yourself: Today I will be grateful for everything I have, I will not focus on things I have and do not want, I will simply feel thankful and joyful for all the things I'm grateful for, all the things I currently have in my life. I do this with everything from having a refrigerator in my kitchen that keeps my food fresh and water cold, to looking at my daughters as their still sleeping, admiring their unique beauty and feeling the love, joy and gratefulness for the simple fact that I have them in my life. You can repeat, and I would encourage you to do this, as many times as you can throughout your day, even if you only have five minutes while your kids are at ball practice. You can do this for anything in your life you feel grateful for. REPEAT. REPEAT. REPEAT.

Chapter Four
Making the Cut

To Whom It May Concern:

Unfortunately, due to unforeseen circumstances we are going to have to let you go. We apologize for any inconvenience.

Have you ever seen a letter like this? It may not be that you've ever received it personally, but I'm sure these are words you've heard before, even if just in movie. Letting go, making cuts, is never easy. It's usually difficult not only for the person getting cut, but also for the person making the cut. This next life practice isn't going to be easy, so it's time to take a deep breath and jump because this step is going to require focus and determination if you're wanting to go to the next level. I can however offer this advice, take this part at your pace, even if you feel like you're moving at the speed of a turtle crawling through mud, it's okay, don't get discouraged or upset with yourself. Cutting people out of your life is never easy and it's important that you let your spirit take charge of this delicate process. Look at it this way, instead of looking at it as cutting people from your life, look at it as releasing people or things that no longer help you grow or contribute to your life. Over half of the people and things you've attached to over your life will graciously leave on their own, you may even realize that the only reason they were still there is because of your efforts to keep them. You may feel reluctant as you start this part of your journey, due to old patterns and old habits, but this releasing or allowing people and things to leave your life, will result in positive outcomes.

By doing this you will also be clearing past relationships that no longer serve any purpose. This will open doors to new relationships and paths that are prosperous and beneficial. I'm not saying you must let go of everyone, I'm saying you must let go of the attachment you have on everyone in your life. People that add quality to your life and receive a quality in their life from you will remain. Not only will they remain, but those relationships will grow and develop with love and compassion for one another. It's a beautiful outcome for everyone involved. People who have applied this and put it in action, including me, have witnessed such a positive result, especially with their children, that words can't come close to describing. It's truly an amazing experience.

Fear plays a big role in this area of spiritual development. Most people are fearful to lose things they have held onto for so long. They attach a sense of who they are to things they own, identifying their selves with materialistic objects, afraid that if they let go, they will be letting go of a piece of who they are. People also get fearful to release other people from their lives. The reasons behind human fear vary substantially; nevertheless, it still boils down to being afraid to making necessary decisions that will better your life and the life of your children.

Your children see what you surround yourself with, people, things, etc. When they grow up, they are likely to follow in your steps to an extent. They can also be influenced by other people you allow around them. This can have both a negative and positive effect, so as you can see this releasing (making the cut) process, is a top priority in spiritual growth.

I have personally put action behind this practice in many areas of my life. I have released attachment to my closest circle, including my children, by releasing this attachment of 'ownership'. Let me be frank, we do not own our children mommas. They are not property. Yes, we birthed them, and they are of our very flesh, and I know the love we feel for our babies is incomparable with all other love, but we still do not have ownership of their lives. They have free will and that free will grows as they grow. By releasing thoughts of ownership (attachment) over our children, we unveil a beautiful process of the deepest love and gratitude. For the fact is, we get to witness and take part in such an amazing life journey with them, we no longer feel as though we must be in control, we are one and can enjoy every moment with them freely.

My children are my life as I'm sure your children are your life. Don't misunderstand what I'm telling you, you don't release your kids to go play unsupervised and say, "I'm practicing not being attached to my kids!" I'm going to repeat this: You simply free your attachment of ownership, example: thinking they should make a certain decision because you think it's the best path and getting angry if they choose another way, that's attachment. You may be thinking, what if I know the path that they are headed toward is destructive? I didn't say to not offer advice or even provide discipline when necessary, children need guidance. Don't confuse teaching right and wrong or protecting your children with releasing attachment. Keep it simple, don't over think the process, it's not something bad. It's to help you grow, to help your children grow and for love to flow more freely without bounds on either end.

When it comes to other people, take your spouse or partner for example. Same process applies here. Release your attachments you may have with them. An example of this may be feeling like you're nothing without them, or you're not sure who you are if you're not with them. That's attachment. If you find yourself trying to change them to suit what you think is best and getting aggravated or mad if they don't conform to your wants. Then you are attached. Let's release all of that, its weighing you down; it weighed me down with my spouse. It's also not fair to them. They are unique in their own way, with their own wonderful qualities. Don't put such a cloud of your attached thoughts over them that you prohibit their light from shining.

I know you may have heard this before, but I'm going to say it anyway, love them for who they are and not what you think they should be. If your main reason for being with them is because you've attached your own identity with theirs (fearful of losing yourself if you don't have them or you're not sure who you are without them in your life), then you need to learn to stand on your own and recognize that your spirit is just as bright as every spirit and doesn't take identity with anyone else. These practices are to help you be able to do that. Love freely, release attachment (any thoughts you have of ownership or control, any expectations you have over what they do or how they act, you must release and allow them to be just as they are), so that you cannot only love them with no judgment, but you can receive that same love. If you put action behind this process, the result will provide the best outcome for not only your life, but theirs also.

Parents. I fortunately had a very easy process in releasing attachment with my parents, we have a strong bond and my mother has taught me most of what I know today with spirituality, she's my personal Eckhart Tolle. Releasing for me came easy when it came to them, because I didn't have a lot of deep-rooted underlying attachments. However, this is not always the case; in fact, I didn't realize that so many people I know and am close with have such a straining relationship with their parents. I have turned to them with ideas and skills to offer you if you too struggle in this area of your life.

I have a close friend that struggled extremely hard in this area of her life. She had blossomed in most every skill of spirituality and had grown immensely in her journey, but when it came to the subject of her parents, especially her mother, she was blocked. Exploring option after option, putting action behind every lesson from every spiritual book she had read and still this 'muck' (issues that are your hardest to overcome) kept rising within every time she spent an extended amount of time with her parents or with her mom. After almost a year of practicing spiritual skills with this lifelong issue, she and I sat down for a heart to heart. I asked her, "Why do you think you keep coming back to this emotion of such discomfort, aggravation and heartbreak?" I asked her what age she envisioned herself, developing this deep pain. Her reply, after deep thought and a process of elimination was, "I see myself at 14, like the 14-year-old in me wants/needs her to say she's sorry for anything she may have done, even if she's not aware of what she was doing. I want her to say she loves me unconditionally and mean every word." There it was, the 'muck' rising to the surface. She was entangled in her own black sticky consuming tar, just like I had been when my 'muck' of facing my past surfaced. This 'muck' must be dealt with before you can release attachment and forgive in the way the spirit intends. I told her that she would probably never receive the heartfelt apology she was searching for and that she would need to overcome this another way.

Almost as soon as I said this, I had an overwhelming feeling to remind her of a love she received from a grandparent, this was a love that was pure, a love she could remember and hold onto. My friend start crying, as did I, she said, "That's right! I did receive the unconditional love I have been searching for from my mom, I just didn't receive it from my mom, but I did get it!" she was so moved by allowing this love she had always had to resurface she was able to move past her block with her mother, although she hadn't gotten what she had sought out for, an apology, she got something more. She received a reminder of a real unconditional love that was bestowed upon her for her whole life. She said, "I had it all along, I was just looking for it in the wrong place." She told me that this allowed her to forgive her mom and release her attachments, attachments of wanting something she'd likely never receive and any other strongholds she was struggling to overcome.

With this releasing attachment (making the cut) she was able to let go of so much she had carried with her most of her life, forgive, and move to the next level of her spiritual self with nothing holding her back in this area. Her relationship with her mother has begun to grow and heal, she no longer is looking for her to provide comfort or apologies, she is accepting her for the person she is and loving her in a way that only a spiritually enlightened person can. Loving the only way you can once attachments are released... Purely without judgment.

There have been many people I know that have carried their own burdens of similar parental issues, this story stood out to me, so I thought it important to include in this book in hopes that if this is your 'muck' you can overcome it.

TIP: Forgiving your parents so that you can make the cut of your attachments and lean to release. Start by digging deep, exploring all memories and past occurrences that may be the 'root of the cause' if there are many, make a list. Explore within yourself until you're settled on the age that these issues began to implant. I want you to practice a skill you've already learned. Forgiveness of Self. Go back to chapter one if you need a refresh. Practice this skill; remember you must first forgive yourself before you can forgive others. Once you have completed forgiveness of self, envision your parent or parents standing before you, I want you to visualize yourself holding a flower between you. Feel only love for your parents as you do this, even if it's just a love for the simple truth that they provided a vessel for you to enter this world, say out loud, I FORGIVE YOU AND I RELEASE MY ATTACHMENTS FOR YOU. Feel love between you as you practice this skill.

These three people or persons are typically your closets relationships, so I have chosen to highlight them; however, there are many other people that you typically know and are involved in your life, you must also release attachment of them. This process is performed and works the same way as with your closest relationships. Ever heard the quote 'Let them go and if they return, they were meant to be there'… guess what, there is truth in that. If you are providing their life with positive qualities and they are providing you with the same thing, then just like law of attraction states, like attracts like, and you will both benefit from having each other or vice versa.

This process includes objects, habits and addictions. Release any attachments you have for your belongings, house, car, clothing, money, etc.…do not identify who you are with these materialistic things. It's fine to enjoy them, be grateful for them and appreciate them, but do not confuse those feelings with an emotional bond that binds you to them. If you have a habit, release your attachment to it. I used to be a nail biter, I felt like I did it subconsciously at times, make yourself aware of your habit and the next time it surfaces replace it with something positive. Instead of biting my nails, I will grab a bottle of water to drink. Retrain your habitual thought pattern. Addictions work the same way; although, may feel more difficult to overcome, you'll have to apply every ounce of your desire to grow spiritually with this process; you'll have to allow your desire for a better life to be more powerful than your addiction.

Here's a common attachment that most people don't even view as an attachment, we view it as a necessity –

MONEY. Money is a big part of almost every human's life. It's almost a requirement. Ask 10 people if they found a genie lamp and got three wishes what those wishes would be? I guarantee at least eight, if not all, say unlimited money! Why? Because we live in a world where money is viewed as a key part of survival, it's viewed as something that will provide a better life. Sure, you can buy a nice house, car and all the materialistic comforts you desire with big bucks, but if this is all a person is supposed to seek, all a person is supposed to achieve in their life on this planet, then riddle me this... Why do wealthy people commit suicide? Why do they suffer from addictions? Why do they suffer from depression? Simple answer: Money doesn't buy happiness.

We have an attachment to money that derives from an unconscious level of fear. It is programmed into our society and we grow up in this world thinking it's a requirement for a happy life. Hate to burst your bubble, but it's not. It can only make your life better if you're happy with yourself, if you're not attached to it and if it's not your sole purpose in life to have it. If you're miserable and rich, then what? What do you do once you've achieved this wealth without seeking spiritual knowledge? And your inner purpose to contribute to mankind has been lost among all the things you've bought to try and fill the gap? You go back to the beginning, you soul search, you find inner peace and start your ever-growing spiritual journey. It must start with this step, the first step of acknowledging that there is a higher power, a higher consciousness. You must take control and begin your own personal journey toward the life you're craving. It's out there, it's waiting for you and everyone else and releasing attachment is just another step on your staircase to becoming your true self, to being spiritually enlightened.

When you release your emotional attachment to someone or something, you have released your expectations and your judgments toward that object. The reason we catch ourselves having the same thoughts we thought we had released, is because our brains have been conditioned to create that thought over and over for a long period of time. Just like my habit of biting my nails or if you twirl a piece of hair while watching tv or check the doors five times to make sure they are locked before going to bed. A habit is when you condition the physical brain to repeat an activity until it becomes automatic. Once you have released a spiritual block or clog, the next process is applying a 're-training' of the brain's thought pattern in that particular area. How do you do this? By understanding that every time you become aware that you're following an old thought pattern then simply say to yourself (to your brain, actually): This is a thought pattern that I'd like to let go of and not create anymore. Then replace those thoughts with a thought pattern or idea that you want to take the place of the old thought. By doing this over and over, every time you catch yourself re-creating those non-productive thought patterns, your brain will start automatically replacing those thoughts with your new thoughts.

When you release your attachments on everything in your life, you're releasing fear and expectations. An important part of releasing is asking anyone who you have an attachment to for their forgiveness. I know this may be a difficult task for some, but by asking someone to forgive you for any hurt or pain you may have caused them in their life and by letting them know you hope they can find it in their heart to forgive you, not only helps them relinquish their judgments they may be carrying against you, but it releases you from any guilt or unnecessary judgments you may not even know that you're carrying within yourself. This act of kindness, by asking for forgiveness, provides a benefit for everyone involved.

REMEMBER: Attachment is a feeling or emotional bond that binds one to a person, thing, cause, ideal, or object. You can control your thoughts and emotions; therefore, you can release your attachments. Releasing attachment is a precondition you must complete before you're able to spiritually love another thing.

I'm going to list a step process that may help you in this 'making the cut' process of your spiritual journey. For my busy moms: This takes about 10 minutes to write down, if you can't go over it immediately, write it down and come back to it later.

1. Make A List
    (Make a list of everyone and everything in your life that does not bring happiness, positive emotions, or quality to your life.)
2. Make A List
    (Make a list of everything in your life that does bring happiness, positive emotions, and quality to your life.)
3. Forgive Yourself
    (Forgive anything you may be feeling negatively about toward people or things in your life. Practice forgiveness of self. Chapter One.)

4. Forgive Them

   (Let go of expectations and release negative attached emotions.)

5. Ask for Forgiveness

   (Go to them and apologize for anything you may have ever done to bring them pain, heartache or discomfort.)

6. Take Time to Heal

   (Meditate and quiet your mind so that it may heal) free guided meditation links are listed at the end of the book.

7. Start Accepting People for Who They Are

   (Release your attachments and expectations.)

8. Practice Positive Thinking

   (Start each day with positive affirmations. Example: I will make the best of this day, I will be kind to myself and others, I will not judge anyone. Today is a good day and I will make positive decisions throughout this day. Think good thoughts that make you happy inside.)

9. Love You for You

   (Show yourself some love! Say to yourself: I love me! Recognize all your wonderful qualities and appreciate all you have within.)

10. Feel Good

    (Let all these good and happy feelings bubble up within you, rising to the surface and replacing any negative thoughts or emotions.)

11. Approaching the Situation

    (Approach each situation that you may encounter with peace, kindness and understanding and the result will be better for everyone. Practice loving the things and people in your life for what they are, without attaching your identity or expectations to them. Control your emotions, your outpour, so that the joy and love you are putting out you can receive. Remember, showing kindness to someone, may change their entire day for the better.)

12. Be Grateful

(Practice feeling gratitude for all you have in your life, for being able to practice these steps, for guidance and spiritual knowledge and for being able to release attachments so that you can experience pure love.)

13. Invest your love in someone who knows how to love you without conditions.

14. Say to Yourself This Truth: It's never too late to love or be loved.

REPEAT. REPEAT. REPEAT.

"Try not to confuse attachment with love. Attachment is about fear and dependency and has more to do with love of self than love for another. Love without attachment is the purest love because it isn't about what others can give you because you're empty. It is about what you can give others because you're already full."

The Minds Journal

Chapter Five
Catch and Release

"Give a man a fish and you feed him for a day. Teach a man to fish and you feed him for a lifetime." – Chinese Proverb.

This next chapter is to help you focus on the negative thoughts you catch and hold onto and how to release and replace them with new positive thoughts. I could've just listed examples of positive thoughts, but I'd rather teach you a practice that constantly allows positive and uplifting thoughts to come into focus, replacing negative thoughts, this practice will be something you can apply for the rest of your life as opposed to something that may only help today.

Let's start by identifying any negative or doubtful reoccurring thought patterns, let these thought patterns become known to you. Writing them down may help you keep track. If you're having trouble recognizing these negative thoughts, then let your emotions guide you on which thoughts don't feel good, the ones that bring about anything that makes you feel negative in any way. Let these thoughts become known to you, take a moment to find the source of where and when these thoughts typically arise. Example: If you don't like your job and every time you wake up for work you think to yourself, I wish I didn't have to work today, or if you start feeling frustration anytime something to do with work comes up, then this would be negative thoughts and emotions you've attached to your job. Another example would be: Your spouse has been in a bad mood these last couple days and keeps snapping at you. You can't think of anything you might have done to be upsetting so your reaction is that you get mad or aggravated that they have chosen you as an outlet, this may even escalate to an argument because you're allowing their outpour to affect you. Then before you know it, when you're thinking of your spouse, while this situation is occurring, you start to feel irritated at all that has been going on, focusing on all your current issues and problems, none of which make you feel good. These would be ideal things to write down. Everyone has their own 'trigger points' so don't feel overwhelmed or frustrated with yourself if your list seems long. This isn't something for you to feel upset over, this is to bring to light all that has you doubting yourself or thoughts that are making you feel bad that keep coming up so that you can practice a skill to help.

I know as a mother, if the kids have had a lot going on or if my two-year-old spends several days running around like she's had five cups of coffee, then it can make me feel extremely tired, so things that normally wouldn't affect me do, there are times that I feel like everything is balancing on me and all I really want is a good nap. It can be overwhelming, so I'd like to take a moment to tell my mommas that are reading. This helps. It helps a lot. It can bring a moment of peace to a day of running around like a chicken with your head cut off, so to speak. So if your day has been a rat race between school drop off, doctors' appointments, target, pick kids up, ball practice, make dinner, help with homework, bath time and story time with kisses goodnight, then before you hit your bed and melt into your pillow, take five minutes. Yes, just five minutes and replace any overwhelming thoughts with this practice I'm getting ready to teach you.

Breathe In. Breathe Out. I want you to close your eyes and breathe in through your nose and out through your mouth. See the breath you're breathing in as white for healing. Cool white healing air. See the breath you're breathing out as reddish brown, this air contains any toxins, hurt, pain, frustration or anything else that may make you feel bad, anxious, stressed or overwhelmed. Feel the tension of the day as it leaves your body. Raise your shoulders toward your ears and release, feeling the tightness in your muscles dissipate. I'd like for you to think of the most negative occurring thought you have currently. (Example: Mine was having doubt I would achieve my inner most desires, saying things to myself when a positive thought or desire would arise: You'll never have that, you're being ridiculous to think you could, be realistic, how do you honestly expect to achieve that?) Think of something you think of often that you wish you could either stop thinking of or stop attaching negativity too. I'd like for you to say to yourself (your mind) I know I keep thinking this because I have always had this thought whenever I do (whatever is causing you to have this thought occurrence, thought pattern) or whenever happens (whatever is upsetting you or bringing about this thought), but it's time to let it go, I'm not going to catch this thought anymore and hold on to it. If I forget and accidently 'catch' it, then I'd like to release it and replace it with (your inner most desire, the thing that makes you feel at your highest level of peace and joy.). Now, you may be asking yourself, "How do I know what my inner most desire is?" Well, I'm so glad you asked.

Close your eyes again. Breathe in and out. I want you to travel deep within yourself and think of the one place on this earth you see yourself being happy, don't attach any thoughts of, I can't afford to live there or I need to keep it realistic, I don't care if you see yourself peaceful on the moon or if it's just the thought of sitting on your porch with a good book and a cup of coffee, feeling the warm gentle breeze upon your skin, just see yourself at the place that makes you feel at your inner most peace and completeness. See this place in detail, if it's the beach, then envision the sand, the ocean, the waves, feel the heat of the sun, smell the salty air, hear the seagulls as they fly overhead. Be There. Think of who is with you, is your mom or dad there? Do you have a partner with you or your children, maybe a pet? Or are you alone, whatever you wish, whatever feels the most peaceful and complete to you. Is the beach crowded or private? Are you walking with the water hitting your bare feet or are you sitting on the warm sand? Do you own a home there or are you just visiting? If you own a home, envision it in detail. The color, the size, the porch, is it beach front or a street back? How many bedrooms? How is it decorated? What does it feel like? I'd like for you to envision this with such detail that in your mind it becomes real. I want you to live in this moment of peace. Let the feeling of peace and completeness consume you as your deepest desire forms into thought. Breathe in and out as you allow this thought to produce peace. Say to yourself: I have nothing to complain about.

Open your eyes. Now tell yourself (your mind) whenever thought arises for whatever reason, I want to let go of my reoccurring negative thought and replace it with this new thought that I have laid out for you in detail.

By the way, you just did it. You thought of something negative that I asked you to recognize as something you think of often and then you applied this skill, I just taught you. You replaced your negative thought with your thought of pure desire that allowed peace to flow through you. Congratulations, doesn't that feel better? I know it did for me; my personal thought of peace is the beach, which is why I chose it for my example to practice. I envisioned every single detail of my perfect day with my family at our cottage style beach home. I didn't attach any thoughts of 'I wish this were real' or 'I want this so bad' I just let my thought and emotion of peace and completeness consume me, which in return made it, for that moment, real. It was real in my mind and had successfully replaced my self-doubting thought pattern. If you continually practice this skill any time a thought surfaces that you wish wouldn't or you find yourself thinking that you wish you could stop going back to this thought, then take some time to replace it with your peaceful thought that you have tucked away for this exact moment. Say those same words to yourself, that you'd like to let it go and replace it with 'this' thought (the thought you've created as its replacement). This will retrain your mind to let go of its past conditioned thought pattern and create a new thought pattern anytime you have one of these occurrences.

This process is truly limitless. You can learn to replace any thought with another. Just make sure the thought you're using as your replacement adds value, quality and benefit to your life. It would be pointless to replace a negative thought with another negative thought. I found this to be one of my favorite and most helpful spiritual tools. It helped me not only form positive new thought patterns, but it made me look at things differently when it came to certain thoughts I had about people. It brought to light, for me, some judgments I was passing on people in my life. Judging was something I wasn't even aware was an issue for me to overcome until I started this process of catch and release. I noticed that I was attaching some of my negative thoughts to things people were doing that I didn't think they should be doing, so I had to recognize this and replace it with a positive thought. The positive thought brought me a more fulfilling emotion whereas the negative thought was only bringing irritation and then anger at myself for thinking I even had a right to judge.

You can also teach this process to your kids. It's worked great with my oldest, my little one is only two so we haven't gotten to practice this skill with her, but my 9-year-old has just started putting this into a conscious act throughout her day. This year has been a little tougher than most for her, she's in a new school and has unfortunately, had her first encounter with some 'not always nice' girls. She's been under some stress with all of this and has experienced having some self-doubt accompanied with negative emotions. When this happens and you're faced with momma bear wanting to come out because kids aren't seeing what you see in this wonderful child of yours, it can make things hard when explaining and helping this issue. So, I turned to meditation, remembering that the higher power is guiding me, mindful parenting skills and the catch and release process. I talked to her about some self-doubt's 'mommy' has had and that everyone at some point usually has their own battle with this issue. I taught her my process and how I overcome this thought pattern and asked her to try it and see if it works for her. We have had many discussions and cuddles accompanied by guided children's meditation and by her putting action behind this catch and release process, the combined efforts are really paying off. She's making great progress and is feeling so much better. If your child is experiencing similar issues or thought patterns, remember that this skill may work for them just as it may work for you.

This process of thought replacement can also help when replacing expectations with intentions.

I'll start by explaining the difference between intention and expectation and how this catch and release process works in this area.

If you have a thought that you want to pick some numbers to play the Powerball, the numbers you pick are 1, 2, 3, 4, 5 with the Powerball the number 6 and you walk into a gas station and buy a ticket with these six numbers written on it. No further thoughts, just six numbers you picked and wanted a Powerball ticket with them on it. You thought of six numbers, you wanted to play them toward the lottery, so you got a ticket and put these six numbers on it, then you have completed your intention. You thought of the numbers, decided you'd play them for the Powerball and bought a ticket. That was your intention. However, if the numbers are drawn and do not match what you have picked and you start to feel upset, you may get so frustrated that you curse and swear to never play again, that's when you know you had an expectation. You picked those numbers so that they would be drawn. You had an expectation on your intention of simply picking six numbers to play for the Powerball. Now, I know your saying to yourself, well duh, why else do you play the lottery if you don't want to hit. That's where this becomes delicate to explain. Your intention was to pick six numbers. You did that. You succeeded with your intention. You picked your numbers and bought your ticket. Your expectation was that the universe was going to show those six numbers as the lottery winning numbers. You attached an expectation which requires the act of someone or something else to help fulfill your desired outcome.

Intentions only rely on you and your actions; they never rely on the actions of anything or anyone else. This is where most people mess up. A lot of times, you know you've attached an expectation because the feeling that comes after the fact. If you feel aggravated, irritated or disappointed with the outcome then you have attached an expectation. If you have an intention of spreading kindness and compassion everywhere go, to everyone you encounter, then let that be your intention without attaching an expectation. Don't be concerned or worry yourself of whether someone is going to be receptive to it, you cannot control other people's reactions or actions. That's not why you're doing it, you're doing it with the pure intention of spreading kindness and compassion. Doesn't that feel better than doing it because you're expecting a certain outcome from it? If you're applying for a new job position, you know if you get that job, the result will be a promotion, but let your intention be that you are going to give the best interview that you can give and feel good about that and then let it go. If you get the job, great, if you don't, then know that the universal energy is going to open a different door for you that may offer a more rewarding result. One more example would be: when you purchase a gift for someone, whether it be for Christmas, Valentine's Day, Anniversary or a just-because gift, your intention should be that you're buying that gift out of the act of pure kindness. The intention of buying that gift is just to show the other person that you're thinking of them and that you care and you feel grateful that they are a part of your life. That's all, it's that simple. If you bought that gift, let's say on Valentine's Day or your anniversary, and your partner did not get you anything in return, then feelings of anger and hurt start to arise, that's an immediate red flag for you to recognize that there was an expectation attached to your intention. Buying the gift is just to let that person know they are important to you, not because you wanted them to buy you something too. Which leads me to my next chapter. Gratitude.

NOTE:

What is Gratitude?

Gratitude is deeper than just being happy for what you have. It's more than saying 'I'm so glad I have a pretty house and pretty things.'

True gratitude goes beyond being happy with your surroundings. It's a feeling that will humble you. It's being satisfied and thankful for everything and for the experience. How do you know you're being grateful? Ask yourself this: Do I feel at peace when I look around me? Do I feel a sense of total humbleness and thankfulness for all that I have?

Gratitude is simply a thankful and humbling state of being. It's being able to appreciate everything without being attached to it.

Attachment takes you out of a state of gratitude and into a state of fear and ego.

Chapter Six
Gratitude

G: **giving** **R**: **receiving** **A**: **abundance** **T**: **thankfulness**
I: **intentions** **T**: **trust** **U**: **understanding** **D**: **discovery**
E: **eternal**

Gratitude. What a powerful word. What makes this word so powerful? What magic it can do, when you're living in a state of gratefulness. Out of all the words that exist, this is one of the most magical. When you shift your mindset, from taking things for granted or not necessarily appreciating things entirely, to being totally appreciative and becoming aware of the value that people and things can add to your life, then you shift your perception of the world around you. Doing this provides a deep sense of joy and humbleness unlike any other emotion.

I'd like for you to do an experiment for me. The next time you're rushing to cook dinner before you have to leave and pick up your other kids and you feel a little tug at the bottom of your shirt, so you look down and your little one is whining and crying wanting attention, instead of saying, "Mommy's busy right now, go play please," step back. Take a breath and turn your stove on low, look at your toddler, look into the eyes of this beautiful little person you brought into this world and think about how little they are, take a moment to think about their age (whether they're 2, 3, 4) however old, they will only be that age for one year out of their whole life. One year out of eternity. They will never be this age again. Take the next 15–30 seconds, give them their sippy and a snack, put their favorite cartoon on, kiss them on the head and now you can go back to your cooking. If they come over again, pick them up, if it's one thing we are good at as mothers it's holding a baby on our hip while still being able to complete almost any task. Basically, what I'm saying is don't lose your temper and get frustrated, don't forget that you can choose your reactions and emotions. Instead of getting aggravated because this moment seems hectic, take those extra seconds and tend to your baby, that won't be a baby forever. The thing you're doing can wait a few seconds.

Doesn't this feel like the best option and response? Feel the gratitude for those little moments bubbling up, instead of letting frustration take over (Catching the emotion of frustration and releasing it, so you can proceed with a calmer response) take control of this moment, be mindful and be grateful for this time you have with your child. Choose to produce a positive outcome with your choice of stepping back briefly. This makes you and your child/children feel better, all the way around. Sometimes, we just need a small reminder of how precious time is; a reminder to be thankful for those little tugs on your shirt. You can always go back to cooking or whatever you're doing, you won't always have an adorable toddler by your side asking for a little attention. Remember, you are their whole world. You're their everything. Don't let everything that's going on in your life become such a focal point that you can't step aside and spare a couple of minutes.

Practicing gratitude for these little moments goes hand in hand with a skill, known to many, as mindful parenting. As with mindful parenting, remembering to pause, step back and choose to approach situations with kindness and understanding, while you wipe down the sharpie scribbled picture on your wall you were just presented with as a 'present for mommy' can feel like an enormous job. It's not always going to be easy for you to remember that there is another approach, especially if you're upset at the F you're staring at on the report card you were just handed, that you know you asked at least 15 times if you could help them study for in the class they've just failed. If you didn't succeed in this practice today, I have fantastic news for you! You get to try again tomorrow. Also, remember to show yourself some compassion, you may not nail it every time, so try, try again. My mom showed me a great point of reference for this skill: Have you ever seen the kid's movie Matilda? (If not, I highly recommend) When you reflect at the end of the day, ask yourself: Were you Mrs. Trunchbull or Miss Honey? That should put things in perspective for you.

TIP: Some little things you can do to show your kids you're grateful for them.

- **Pack A Lunch Note**
  This is a big thing at our house, my 9-year-old loves her 'napkin notes' she receives on her lunchtime. It takes

almost no time out of my day to write on her napkin, 'I can't wait till you get home, hope your day is going awesome, I love you, sunshine,' and for a moment, even though were apart, she can feel my presence. It's a simple task that can make all the difference in your child's day at school.

- **Clean Isn't A Word They Know Yet**

  Remember that your kids are kids and what do kids like to do? Kids like to be messy, let them! Well, let them be messy at times. I understand the constant need for cleanliness, trust me, but it's ok to let them play as hard as their little heart's desire at times without being wiped down in between. If it's not hurting anyone, then just let them play, heck, join them if you'd like! Be grateful for the messy time and the shower that follows!

- **Be A Kid, With Your Kid**

  When was the last time you ran through a yard with fairy wings on, swinging a wand around to stop the evil trolls from entering your secret garden and stealing your fairy dust? When was the last time you had to fake fight an entire ship of pirates during your bath time to protect your gold doubloons? Let your imagination shine again, let it shine with your kids. Play with them; take the time to show interest in their fun filled world of imaginary games.

- **Include Them**

  I know that alone time is important and I'm not suggesting you never have it, but make sure you're also taking time to include your kids in things you love to do, introduce them to the big world, they will soon be fully emerged in, it's almost like 'becoming older orientation' and it will help them be more comfortable when they do start having their own adventures. It will also introduce them to a side of you they may not see often, a relaxed you that has nothing on the schedule today.

- **Laugh Often**

  Laughing is so important, it's a natural stress reliever; use it as much as possible. Almost anything can make kids laugh, so the next time you find yourself riding in your car, 10 minutes from home and no has made a peep. Make a crazy face, tell a joke, it won't take much to get a laugh out of them, but it will make all the difference in the trip

  I was going to stop on the laugh tip after that sentence, but I must add this for those having a hard time finding something to laugh about...

  So, this just happened. I'm sitting at my desk, writing this book, as my two-year-old watches a cartoon. She walks up to me with, what looks like chocolate on her fingers and it appears she's also wiped it on her shirt; however, with closer examination and a small whiff, this chocolate in question is poo. That's right, she's stuck her hand down her diaper and pulled out a nasty, smelly little surprise, just for me! I've decided to write about this little incident because it made me LAUGH! I also thought it would be perfect for telling you this: I could've gotten justifiably frustrated at this incident, she's just had a bath, those clothes are, well, were clean and I'm trying to write, but why do all that, when all I really should be doing is laughing and being grateful that she didn't eat her own natural 'chocolate'.

- **Sing and Dance**

  Dance with your kids! It's fun! Be Silly! My daughter and I have this little thing we love to do called 30 second dance party. Take some time every day or every other day, even if it's once a week, take time and have yourselves a '30 second dance party'. I've been in the middle of doing the dishes and I'll take a moment, stop everything and yell throughout the house, "30 SECOND DANCE PARTY!" My girls run to me and we break it down, no music playing, goofy dance moves for 30 seconds. There's no reason for this other than simply having fun. My kids love it. It shows them I was thinking of them and brings nothing but fun and happiness to that moment. Dancing is a great way to express happiness. Same goes with singing, sing your heart out. Sing to them, sing with them. Make it a game. Hum a tune to your kids and have them guess what song you're singing, then have them do it to you. Music is therapeutic, expressive and even magical. It can provide the words you may lack, explore it with your kids. I'm not sure why when we become adults it seems like fun packs a bag. We sometimes lose that playful side we had as kids. Bring it back. Your kids can help you in doing that if you'll let them. Sing and dance with them anytime you have the chance.

- **Decision Time**

  Allow your kids to make some decisions of their own. Example: My niece has her own personal style and it's important to her that she likes the clothes she wears. My sister-in-law, who has three kids, a dog, a spouse and full-time job, doesn't have a lot of extra time to let her pick her clothes before school or disagree about the ones she may have laid out, so to help herself with this dilemma she has Veto Sunday. On veto Sunday she and my niece lay out the upcoming week outfits and accessories, my niece has veto power on this day only, if she doesn't like it, that's her only day to change the planned outfit, otherwise, she's wearing it. This allows her to make her own decision on something that's important to her. Allowing kids to make their own decisions helps them with responsibility and lets them know that you value their opinions and trust that they can decide things for themselves.

- **Teamwork**

  Teach them through teamwork. Example: when it comes to housework use this motto: if you help me with dinner or dishes, then I have time to do something fun with you. Simple things like that can make all the difference in the big picture. Your kids won't remember the chores. They will remember the time you took afterward to play with them. That's what they'll be grateful for.

  These tips are to help you in showing your children that you're grateful you have them, grateful you're their parent. Actions can speak louder than words and sometimes just hearing 'you make me happy' or 'I'm proud of you' isn't enough. So, if you start feeling stuck in your efforts, try these tips. They can help guide you in showing gratitude for your children. Showing gratitude for your children also helps them show it toward each other and to other people they know and will meet throughout their lives. Make sure you give them opportunities to show acts of kindness in their own way. Have them help each other with their homework and chores, they are each other allies in this world and expressing gratitude will strengthen their bond.

Gratitude is more than a feeling of 'I'm really glad I was able to catch this sale' or 'I'm glad I have this house.'. Gratitude is a deeper sense of appreciation, it's not a surface emotion, it's not 'I'm glad I have money to buy this or that' it doesn't leave when the new wears off. Materialistic things can bring temporary happiness, but a true gratitude, a humble feeling of gratitude, is infinite, it doesn't go away. It's not 'I'm so glad I got that shirt' it's being grateful that you have clothing to cover your body. It's a deep appreciation that goes beyond the surface. It's not being grateful because your surroundings are beautiful, it's everything is beautiful because you are grateful.

'It's not happiness that brings us gratitude. It's gratitude that brings us happiness.'

– quoteambition.com

There are many ways you can experience true gratitude daily. When you open your eyes in the morning feel gratitude within, that your eyes opened so you will be able to see throughout this day. Walk through your home and appreciate that you have a roof over head. Feel the deep appreciation at your core. If you're a stay-at-home mom, or if you just don't have to work because your spouse provides you with your home, car, etc.... Instead of saying thank you for my house and car and nice things, feel the gratitude for your partner that they work to provide you with this lifestyle, appreciate that they care enough about you to give you this comfort. Or if you work, be grateful you have a job that enables you to provide it for yourself and your family. Be truly grateful. No matter how little or how much you have in this world, there is always, always something to feel grateful for. This practice is humbling in such a way, that it's hard to describe. Some of you may be surprised to learn you weren't truly experiencing deep appreciation or deep gratitude for your life and all that's in it. It's easy to say, I'm happy for this and I'm thankful for that. Applying true gratitude requires action behind your thoughts of, things you're glad you have.

TIP: Try some of these tips that may help you practice experiencing true gratitude. These are things I have personally done and still do daily.

- Set your timer five minutes early in the morning. I know that most of you, if you're like me, only do this normally so that you can hit snooze at least once, but I'd like for you to pause on the extra five minutes of sleep, go ahead and wake up. As you open your eyes, feel appreciation and allow the feeling of gratefulness to rise in you. Feel grateful that you're awake, that it's a new day, that today you get a fresh start. Approach this day with the thought: You will never get a chance to have this day again, today is today, you can't experience it tomorrow, so be grateful for this day and make it the best day you can.

- Another thing you may like to try is appreciating your home. Walk around your home and look at every detail of it. Look at your decorations, look at your light fixtures, look at your furniture, look at everything you have in your home, including the actual structure of the home itself. Think of all it provides for you. Warmth, shelter, comfort, serenity, a place for your family, allow that deep appreciation to bubble up, it goes beyond the surface. I want you to truly feel the gratitude of the fact that you have this home that provides all that it does for you and the people within it. Say thank you out loud if that helps, you can express thankfulness to the universe for all the things you have in your life at any point in this process, just express it from an honest and deep place within where you can feel true gratitude.

- Last thing: Feel grateful for you, your body. Look at your hands, arms and legs. Feel your lungs pump air in and out without you telling them to do so. You are a living miracle. If you have not one materialistic thing in this world, you still have you. You're a brilliant masterpiece. Be grateful for every organ, every bone, every breath, every heartbeat. FEEL grateful for you.

"Gratitude opens the door to the power, the wisdom, the creativity of the universe. You open the door through gratitude."
Deepak Chopra

Chapter Seven
Hello?

Hello?
Are you there?
Are you there?
Is there an echo?

Why yes, there most certainly is. You may even be wondering how an echo can be related or have anything to do with this book, but echoes and ripples are amazingly important components when living a spiritual path of enlightenment. In this chapter I'll be explaining how your ripples and echoes effect your daily life and effect those around you. Yep, that's right! RIPPLES AND ECHOES! So, hold on to your bloomers because we're diving in headfirst!

Have you ever skipped rocks? When I was a kid, I remember my grandpa showing me how to skip rocks across water. "The flatter the rock the better," he'd say, as he showed me the perfect way to hold the stone and with a flick of the wrist. It would release and skip across the top of the water. As the rock hit the water it would make tiny ripples at the center and grow into larger ripples that extended outward from the point of contact. When you're feeling negative emotions, such as anger, hurt, or aggravation, then just like the stone in the water, you're creating your own ripples. Only your ripples don't just make tiny waves in water, they extend from you; they become your outpour and effect the people around you. Whatever is in your ripple is in your energy, in your 'personal space' and whoever is near you will sense that. It works just like the stone that makes the waves, only in energy form. Your inner emotions ripple from you and extend, echoing outward. Whoever is near your energy field is somewhat subject to your vibes; your echoes. This is a big deal. It can affect so much. I know because I've seen and felt this firsthand.

I envision myself on my spiritual path as me riding this beautiful white horse alongside the beach, just me and this majestic horse. This is a visualization that helps me in keeping focus, because I am easily distracted, in fact I joke and tell my mom at times when I think of this visualization it feels as though my foot is in the stirrup and I'm being pulled alongside this horse through the sand, in other words, barely hanging on. When I allow things to pull my focus away from my intended spiritual path or don't allow myself the necessary time to have moments of silence, moments of peace, moments of reflection and time to study, I start to feel chaotic and frazzled. This creates a sort of downward spiraling ripple that is felt not only by me, but my family. I've noticed if my ripples are filled with this chaotic, busy, overwhelming feeling that it has a huge effect on my kids, husband and family. Negatively.

When we feel stressed or overwhelmed it can, at times, be forgotten that we know any spiritual knowledge or spiritual tips that help deal with circumstances like this.

We get caught up in the moment and sink into emotional chaos that has no structure, no light at the end of this sink hole. This is exactly what I'm talking about with ripples and echoes.

When you ripple down into this sink hole, your echoes become infused with its chaotic nature. This infusion penetrates your energy field and the echoes that project from you create negative vibes. If you do not stop this as soon as you become aware of what's happening, the effects can be many to repair. I, personally, tend to get 'caught up' with certain things that may seem exciting in the now. I can take spontaneous a little too far sometimes. Some of that is a good thing, but if you take something that may require more time to be laid out and you rush it, then you may be faced with problems. When I do this and get toward the end of the situation and my puzzle pieces that I've rushed in don't quite fit like they should, I start to allow frustration and out of balance energy to flow through me. It starts as small ripples and then gets larger and larger with every ounce of focus it receives, every ounce of energy I allow it to consume of me.

This echoes outward toward my family, the closest people to me. I have noticed when this is happening my husband and I start arguing, or disagreeing on things and the peace between us becomes disturbed. My children notice this also and it ripples to them, making them feel aggravated that their parents are not getting along. My oldest at times has expressed stress toward me in these situations, for my ripple has created a negative echo that she has been in contact with and has in turn effected how she is feeling. This is just one example of how allowing something that's off track with the spiritual journey to throw you off your horse and cause disruption, cause negative ripples and echoes.

EXERCISE:

When something starts to pull you off track and you start to feel yourself slipping into emotions of discomfort, aggravation, frustration, overwhelming stress, anxiety and so on... I'd like for you to try something with me. I'd like for you to press stop. Make yourself aware of what is happening and STOP everything. Ask yourself:

Where this feeling is coming from?

What happened that's causing this feeling?

Do a retrace: Trace back through the ripples and get to the core of the emotion, the center point of contact. Study it; study the situation that you've traced back to. Then choose to look at it differently than you are right now. Look at it with peace, instead of a negative emotion. I'm asking you to allow your spirit within to rise and allow the inner peace within you to be stronger than any negative emotion you're feeling. There is another way to look at every situation. There is a peace that can replace the other feeling. Just like the upset emotion that has risen, so can the peace. As you've already learned, you can control your emotions; control them here in upsetting situations. Become aware that you've stepped in quicksand, stop, look around for a branch to grab onto and pull yourself out. I'm saying look for peace to grab onto and then allow it to pull you from chaos.

Approach situations that can cause a break in the spiritual flow with compassion, all things that are negative are simply things that haven't been put into alignment. They are lost. If you allow yourself to submerge into the unenlightened things and situations that arise in life, without allowing your spirit and personal enlightenment to shine through, you too can become lost. So, it is in these circumstances that you will be able to practice your tools of spiritual knowledge and enlightenment to their fullest. You will have to be the light amongst the darkness.

When you start changing your approach to compassionate and peaceful, you will begin changing your ripples. This changes your echoes that are vibrating from you. Your energy that surrounds you will generate what you are infusing into it, peace and compassion. Whoever you encounter will be stepping into this vibe you've surrounded yourself with. It's quite simple if you step back and think about it. Would you rather be around someone that's nice, emitting love for all in a calm approach or would you rather be around someone that's frustrated, emitting chaos and aggravation? Apply this to yourself. Emit Positive Ripples and Echoes.

TIP: Remember What You Put Out, Is What You Get Back

If you're yelling at your kids to do clean their room, pick their shoes up, or 'hurry you're going to be late' and you find them getting an attitude with you quite often, they may be eating from the bowl you've filled with aggressive tone and attitude. I know it can be frustrating when you told them last night to put their homework in their backpack and when you walk out the door, they turn back to get it because they didn't listen, but do yourself and them a favor and don't yell. You can express your point without screaming. Raising your volume can raise the entire house volume, keep it on as normal level as possible so things don't become more chaotic then necessary. Try your best in moments of frustration to make your point in a calm way.

Chapter Eight
Leggo My E.G.O.

Ego. External Glitch of Oneself.

I'm fat and I wish I looked like Jennifer Aniston.
I have the nicest house in my neighborhood and the nicest car. I bet people think I'm rich.

I hope someone tells me I look beautiful today. That will make me feel good about myself.

I'm not too concerned with his personality, if he's hot, I can overlook that.

I'm not as good as her because she's prettier and dresses nicer than I do.

Oh, my goodness, why would someone wear that, don't they know how awful that looks?

Why would they let someone treat them like that?
These are all judgments, judgments toward oneself, judgments toward others. Why are these our thoughts? Why do other's think this? Is it a form of worldly conditioning or insecurities? How do we stop doing this?

I've read many books of spiritual awareness that speak about the ego. The place where all judgments and 'glitches' originate. I've read about killing the ego, vanishing the ego or separating yourself from the ego. I've read these things and no matter what practice comes along with doing these processes I still find myself at these thoughts:

How do you kill something that's in you?

How does something that's always been with you truly vanish?

How can I separate one part of myself from another part of myself?

I'm not saying these practices and teachings aren't the right path for some, but they were not the right path for me. I thought it was difficult for me, personally, to grow beyond my egoic state of mind from that starting point. I have found that it was much easier to look at the ego **(Dictionary: Ego. A person's sense of self-esteem or self-importance)** as something we carry within us that isn't balanced, something that isn't at its full potential of spiritual awareness. It helped me to understand that like so many other parts of me, the ego was just something I had been conditioned to believe was who I am, and like all the other parts of me that weren't as they should and could be, it would need balanced, it would need enlightened. The ego would need to be healed.

Healing the ego takes constant and consistent effort. You must commit that you no longer what to derive your state of being from the egoic place. I know that for me, this process is ongoing even into my current being. I still at times, find myself either passing judgments and doubts on myself or saying things like, "Wonder why someone would wear that." If I see what I view as an unsavory outfit on another person. First off, why do we think it's ok for us to view, what probably made someone else happy as they were staring back at their reflection that morning, as something good or bad, ugly or pretty? Is their hairstyle, outfit or choice of anything they have on affecting your life, is it hurting you? I'd like for you to ask yourself that if a negative thought about someone else's appearance pops into our head. Control the thought, visualize it in front of you and ask yourself that question. Let me tell you about an incident that happened:

My mom has a friend who attends church. My mom's friend was explaining to her how she felt offended by an outfit that someone else had worn to Sunday school. She said it was too revealing and not appropriate for church. After the friend had went on for oh, somewhere around ten minutes, she asked my mom, "What do you do in situations like that?"

My mom replied, "Situations like what?"

Her friend said, "How do you go up to someone and tell them that what they're wearing is inappropriate for Sunday school?"

This conversation leads to these next questions:

1. Are you saying the person should not have worn the outfit because it offended you?
2. What if what they had on made them feel pretty?
3. What if they put the outfit on that morning, looked in the mirror and it made them feel beautiful?
4. Do you think that someone shouldn't wear what they want because of how it made you feel, because you happened to feel offended?

Or should they have worn it because of the way it made them feel?

What if someone's having a bad day and they pick out an outfit, hairstyle, etc. that makes them feel better, that makes them feel happier that day or what if they simply don't know any better and they are just doing the best they can. Regardless of the reason they are not in the wrong. Whoever is passing the judgment is making a choice to place an opinion on someone when really, someone else's opinion of you, or your opinion of someone else is neither of your business.

The number one reason why we shouldn't judge, the reason judging is so damaging and can create hurt to everyone involved:

Judging accomplishes nothing. Nothing. It's a complete waste of time and energy. It does not add any value to your life or the other persons. It is totally non-beneficial for everyone. Here's why:

The energy you're using to feed those judgmental thoughts could be used to send a more beneficial thought to your fellow human being. Instead of placing judgmental thoughts toward them, why not replace that with peace and joy. Use your energy in a positive way and say, I hope peace and joy come into their life. If you run into someone having a bad day or someone that seems to always be hateful and unpleasant, control your thoughts, quiet your mind and send a positive flow their way. Use your outpour and energy to uplift someone else. Send this thought out: I hope their spirit rises to the surface and leads them into a positive direction that helps benefit their life.

Stop the judging. Stop the negativity. Be the change. Start only wishing the best for other humans. Keep peace in mind.

Release any animosity you may feel toward judgments others pass on you. Keep in mind that you cannot change what someone is currently doing, thinking or applying in their life as their routine or the lifestyle they choose. Free will is in play here. We all have it. All you can do is make the choices for yourself to not allow it to affect you, not allow it to penetrate your awareness. You cannot allow others to slow down your growth. Instead what you do is make your energy/vibration stronger in hopes that it will allow them to feel peace in your presence. Now, whether they allow your peaceful outpour to uplift them is again, their choice, but you can find comfort in knowing that you did all you could on your end to make the best and most beneficial decision for everyone.

Putting these thought replacement exercises into action brings so much peace to life. For me, it's become a basic instinct, I look at it as simple as choosing to be the best person I can toward someone else or wasting my energy not being the best. Sometimes it just gets crowded in our minds and we let what everyone else is doing rub off onto us.

Listen ya'll, this is all simple and basic. The reason people complain that have tried to change and tried to learn ways to do better or make changes to themselves and it hasn't worked for them is because it can be hard. Not hard to learn and comprehend what to do, but people can tend to be lazy in their efforts. So, having to apply this knowledge to your life, to make a change within, to be conscious that you must be consistent and always apply everything you're learning about spiritual awareness to yourself and life every day, seems like too much or too hard. It boils down to how bad you want it.

By doing this exercise, applying non-judgment and healing your ego, you're allowing a block in the spiritual flow to release and open. You're allowing for a better use of your time and energy. It's also allowing for a more positive result in the way you perceive the world in which you live.

Make a conscious choice every day of your life to not allow an egoic state of mind to control you today. Be the awareness behind your egoic thoughts and choose to replace them with thoughts that are beneficial to you and to people around you. Start today, start right now, you have an opportunity every day to be a better person this day than you were the last.

TIP: Remember to stand strong in your efforts of making the choice to heal your ego and to stop judging. Don't let friends or outside forces that are beyond your control to allow a halt in your growth with this process. Tell yourself anytime you feel like you are not doing the best at this as you want or could be, whisper to yourself these words:

I am learning and growing every day. I will not judge or place any opinions on others or myself. I will not allow others to affect me or how I feel. I am allowing my ego to heal and become balanced with my spirit.

Today I will be better that I was yesterday.

What is the difference between an Observation and Judgment?
When you make an observation, you're stating something that just is, without emotional attachment or opinion. Judgment has an emotional attachment or opinion on the observation.

Chapter Nine
Show Yourself

Come Out, Come Out, Wherever You Are

"Mom, did you just poop your pants?"

The question my nine-year-old daughter asked me last Christmas Eve on our way home from a very large dinner, where I may or may not have overstuffed myself.

"Yep, sure did," was my reply. As if I could've denied it at this point anyway.

I tried with all I had to make it home before this accident became inevitable. I was so embarrassed to call my father-in-law, who happened to live the closest to where the accident occurred and ask him if I could use one of his bathrooms. I opted for the toilet he literally has against his wall in the garage with no walls to hide it. I thought I could get to it quicker and avoid seeing his relatives that were visiting for Christmas dinner. Since all he had to do was open the garage door, I assumed this would be my best option, I could just run in, easy peasy.

Umm no. No, it wasn't. So, here it is in a nutshell.

I spent my last Christmas Eve partially naked, yes, almost naked because the clothing I was wearing had poop on it, not sure how poop got on my shirt, but nevertheless, it did. So, partially naked on a toilet against a wall in my father-in-law's garage, with the garage door open and cars passing by rather closely I might add because, oh yeah fun fact, he lives almost directly beside a heavily trafficked main road and has zero front yard, while my nine-year-old laughs hysterically as she holds a towel in front of me so people can't watch this drama unfold. We laughed all the way home, with the windows rolled down to air out the car. Oh, the Christmas Joy… #momlife.

Now, you're probably asking yourself, why is this story relevant to this book? Here's why, it's relevant to this chapter! Show yourself is about letting it all hang out, it's about showing your true self, the good, the bad, the funny and embarrassing unique you! So, what if that story is embarrassing, it's me and it's something my whole family has laughed about repeatedly. But that's okay! Just because something may seem embarrassing doesn't make it shameful, learn to laugh at those moments because I can promise your life will not be without them. I hope by now in reading this book you have learned that you are amazing, that your spirit is amazing and that you can do and achieve amazing things. Now it's time to take a chapter to encourage and teach you how to let yourself shine. Let all the qualities you have come out and show the world the beautiful you.

Every spirit/human being on this planet has a purpose. Some people spend their whole lives either not seeking truth, ignoring truth, being afraid of change or just being lazy about making changes to who they are. We each have moments and little things that have happened along the way to help mold us, help make up our personalities. I'm showing you me with this book, I'm telling you about my moments, sharing with you all my deepest, hardest, trying moments. All my embarrassing, I can't believe I'm an adult and that happened moments. I'm teaching you the skills I've learned and used that have helped me grow spiritually as a person, as a parent, as a friend, as your fellow human being. I'm laying it all out on the line for you, with one purpose. To help. I want to help you grow spiritually in every way I can so that you can find your purpose and have a more fulfilled life. I'm catering to my busy moms because I am a busy mom and I'm writing about what I know. I don't have a PHD, I didn't graduate college. I am a small town, southern, stay at home mom. I've never lived more than an hour from my hometown. I married my high school boyfriend and was pregnant at 19. I'm not sitting at a fancy desk having an assistant write my every word. I'm just your average citizen. I have a great hard-working husband that I wouldn't trade for the world and together we have two amazing bright and beautiful daughters. We live paycheck to paycheck and save what we can. No fancy house, no vacation homes, no luxury bank account or limitless credit cards.

I'm telling you this because I want you to know that it doesn't matter who you are or where you come from, you can do this! This will help you find fulfillment and purpose in this busy fishbowl we call life. I was having some great days, some good days, some okay days and some bad days and I thought, I want all great days. I want no doubt. I want more. So, I reached back into my memory vault and pulled out that conversation with my mom, the one she had mentioned some time back about her spiritual journey and how she was applying it to her life and seeing real results.

Thus, my journey began. I immediately started downloading audiobooks of Eckhart Tolle, Deepak Chopra and Tony Robbins, grasping all I could on my drives to work and at breaktimes. I eventually discovered Joe Dispenza and many more that teach about spiritual awareness. I even found videos on Netflix that confirmed what I was learning to be exactly what I felt it to be. Truth. Truth of life. Universal truth. I studied and studied some more, then I had my second child and life went from one kid to what felt like ten kids. My time was more limited so I started searching for quick solutions, quick tips I could grasp so that my growth could continue. There were none. Nothing was coming up that didn't require at least 45 minutes of attention. Other than quick meditation videos or podcasts, I was either going to have to ask my mom to watch my kids so I could read or push it back until time opened. I didn't want to do either, so guess what happened? I put it to the universal energy. I said out loud to the higher power, show me a path, guide me in the direction I need to go in order to continue growing and contributing. I'll never forget it, I was driving in my car singing to the radio with my oldest daughter and a title of a book popped in my head: Growing Spiritually with Schedules, Spouses, Toddlers and Preteens. I immediately called my mom and said, "You may think this sounds off the wall, but I'm going to write a book."

For this next process, I want the motto: No shame in my game to be your mantra. You've spent the last however many days, reading and applying these things you've read to you and your everyday life, now is the time to show off. Shake any self-doubt off to the side and let this person that's allowing the spirit to guide them come out. All the good you've been feeling within is ready to take on the world. Let's do this.

This process will require you to stay focused on your purpose or purposes, being true to who have you become and not allowing others' judgments or opinions of you to affect who you are and how you feel about yourself. Some may say things that are hurtful. Some may say nothing, but you have the thought of self-doubt in their presence, feeling as though they are judging you as you stand before them. Take the skill you've already learned of 'catch and release' let those negative thoughts go and say to yourself: Their opinion of me is none of my business. Then let it go. You will never control someone else's thoughts; they must be willing to make changes within to be a better person, just like you're doing! Be careful not to allow them to pull you back into their negative outpour. Stand strong, stand proud of the enlightened form you have now become. Say encouraging things to yourself throughout your day if you start to feel negative. I found myself looking in the mirror at times, saying: This is the new me, I have allowed and am allowing a great transformation, it doesn't matter if people refuse to see it, I see it and I know I'm a better person today than I was than I was yesterday and tomorrow I'll be better than today. Be confident in this practice. It's perfectly fine if you struggle at times, you will, and you shouldn't expect to be perfect. We are students of the higher consciousness, always learning. When you think you know everything is when it's time to learn even more. Go ahead and pat yourself on the back, it's time for everyone to meet you.

How do you feel right now? Nervous? Excited? Not sure? That's ok, this is a new process. I'd like for you to pick out something to wear today, release all thoughts you have about it, don't be concerned with brands or if someone else will like it, nothing like that. I just want you to pick out an outfit that makes you FEEL happy. That makes YOU feel good. Put it on. You're wearing it today. Now, look at yourself in the mirror and repeat after me: **I'm allowing my spirit to shine today, I feel good and I like the new me.**

Once your outfit is picked out, repeat this same process of hairstyle and makeup, jewelry, etc.…does this make me feel good? No judgments. Release those feelings of 'so and so wore this, so I want to too', you can't be anyone else and I don't want you to be, there's only one you. How you feel about yourself is all that matters. So, put yourself together in the way that makes you feel good.

If you eat breakfast, I'd like for you to approach your meal with this thought. Will this make me feel good? Is it good for my body? Will this provide my body with nutrition to help me be the best I can be today? If not, try and find something that will, replace your thoughts of this tastes delicious with thoughts of nurturing your body. Once you've settled on the food, take a moment and feel grateful for your morning so far. You have clothing on your body and a meal on your plate, that's more than some have ever had, feel the gratitude rise and welcome it with a smile. You're shining! Let's continue.

Your day is now full steam ahead, whether you're getting the kids up or leaving for work, you're about to enter another person's outpour. The people around you have ripples of their own and you're exposed to them throughout your day, so approach each moment of this day with the thought that your positive ripple, your high-spirited outpour will be strong, impenetrable and help increase negative ripples you may encounter in a positive way. You're letting yourself shine. This is awesome. Walk through this day confident in your new-found knowledge, your journey ever stretching before you, you should be proud of what you're learning and putting action behind. It's not easy making changes to who you always thought you were, and it takes constant effort to remain centered in a chaotic world but look at you! You're doing it!

SPEED BUMP! Something happened that just threw you off track, call from school to pick up an upset tummied 4th grader or your boss just informed you you'd be working this Saturday, which means no camping trip. Great. Old familiar starts to rise and the old you would get mad, aggravated, worried, frustrated, immediately anxious. STOP. That's habitual thought patterns and emotions that you're used to coming up like emotional vomit. This is the new you, remember. You've studied and practiced all you need to be equipped for this moment. Step back and replace your thoughts now. You've got this. So, you have to work this weekend, not what you wanted I know, but go with it, who knows someone else that's working this Saturday may benefit from being around your positive energy, when you get home you can re-plan a fun trip! So junior has an upset tummy, clear your worry and send energy out of comfort until you can wrap your arms around your little, then infuse your positive feel-good ripple into them, visualize healing and comfort energy flow from you to them.

Don't expect to not have moments that aren't necessarily in alignment. You will have these consistently through your life because not everyone on this planet is studying spiritual awareness. It's your job to show what you're doing, to use what you know, so that it will have a positive effect. You're changing the course of your life and the life of those close to you for the better.

Chapter Ten
Did I Join the Circus?

Ring. Ring. Ring. "Poison control, how can we help you?"

"Hi, my two-year-old just ate an orange highlighter and I need to know what to do."

True Story.

Is this a balancing act or am I juggling too much at once? Sometimes life and motherhood can have you feeling like you're a one-woman circus act. I don't know about you, but one day in my life could make you feel like you ran a 35K with no breaks. When it comes to adding anything on top of my overly planned days, I'm typically immediately seeing how far I can 'push it back' or if there is anytime I can squeeze it in later. Additional tasks are just not something I like discussing, unless the word vacation is involved. So when my mom started talking with me some years back about this spiritual knowledge she was obtaining through different books and teachings and how much better she was becoming as a person and all the wonderful differences she was seeing in her life, I thought, that's really awesome for you mom, but I just don't have time to read a lot or watch videos and stuff. Is there something quick I can just pick up? Like an all-in-one that covers the basics to get me started. There is now! Woot Woot! And what's more, you're over halfway through! Go You!

Sometimes I feel like one crazy momma. By the end of the week there are times that I feel like I can't do one more thing or I'm just going to go kaput! My grandma once told me that one kid is one kid and two kids are like having one hundred, let me tell ya. This is true, so true. My kids are complete opposites, in fact there are times my littlest is running all over the house, throwing folded clothes, that haven't been put up yet, everywhere and screaming all the while and my oldest will look at me and say, "geez, I never was that rowdy." And it's true, she wasn't, but I wouldn't trade their unique and completely opposite personalities for the world. The key for me has been calming my mind in the chaos of parenting, learning patience, and taking time to enjoy my kids, instead of feeling frustrated with how little time is in one day, frustrated with cleaning up stepped on crumbs in the floor fifteen times and constantly saying, 'don't do that' and 'no, stop'.

If you're reading this and thinking to yourself, story of my life, (Insert 'girl with her arm raised up' emoji) I want you to know that I'm here to help, if you'll let me. I thought my youngest daughter was beginning to think the only words I knew where no and stop. My oldest daughter was complaining that she felt like I spent more time with her little sister. It was frustrating and hard for her to grasp the concept, since she's only nine, of why her two-year-old sister received a little more time because she required constant care. They don't get it; all they see is mommy is with my sibling more than she is with me. It appears unfair to them and explaining doesn't do anything, in my experience. I did a lot of reading and soul searching before I came up with my own little cocktail of solutions that have made an impact for the better in our lives.

I replaced no, stop.

I know that this may sound insane. We heard this when we were kids and it just seems normal to say no non-stop to your over curious toddler, but I was introduced to another way that feels better and works better for my family.

Replace no with, that's not the best decision or you shouldn't do this because... (followed by the reason they shouldn't do whatever they are doing).

Why is saying no something I'm choosing to include in this book:

Saying no without a reason or just hearing no, all the time, can put doubt in the subconscious. So, when they are older and try to make choices it creates a block without them even being aware of why they have a fear or doubt about something. Teaching them to think about their choices and the consequences their choices, bring, better equips them for future choices and allows them to think freely about their choices. That's why it's better to tell them to either think about the action they are about to do or let them know that the action they are about to make may not be the best decision for them due to the consequences that it could cause. Telling them to stop and quit over and over doesn't allow them to think about their choice or consequence. It only tells them no with no explanation why. It ultimately causes them to not think on their own about the choices they are making.

This has been a real effort for me to put into practice. I have an extremely active toddler at home that is constantly grabbing this and that. She literally growls at me if I take something from her that she wants. My husband jokes and calls her our little sour patch kid, because she'll do something that's 'not the best choice' like throw a piece of wooden fake food at your head, and follow it up with kisses and hugs, he says first she's sour and then she's sweet. So, saying no was like I said earlier, my go-to option. I've really had to put effort behind this process, but I can honestly say that I'm seeing better results. She's stopping before acting, for the most part, she seems to be putting thought behind her actions. Not all the time, but enough for me to notice. I also feel better saying, "That's not the best choice sweetheart," and following it up with a reason, it feels like more of a mindful response. Plus, she knows, that I know, more words than. NO. Now! It's a win, win in my book. Try it out. You may be surprised, like I was, at the result.

Patience: not a skill I have been super great with. I would go as far as to say this was top three hardest 'unbalanced' parts of me I had to smooth out. It didn't take much to jump in my elevator and hit every button on the panel. It was a thin layer before I'd begin to crack under pressure. When it came to practicing patience, I used mediation. Specifically, guided meditation. I'll list several links at the end of the book of guided meditation (FREE videos) for the ones I used to overcome this specific issue. I basically had to quiet the chatter long enough to get clarity.

We spend so much time asking, asking, asking, wondering why this and why that, always seeking for answers, that sometimes we forget that in order to receive an answer, at least one that's clear, we must quiet our minds.

I kept asking the higher power for ways to help me with my patience and then I would get aggravated that I felt like nothing was coming through, but I wasn't allowing it. I was so busy searching for an answer that I was blocking the one right in front of me.

Be Quiet.
Take quiet time.
Quiet your thoughts.
Quiet your chatter.

Listen and give time for answers to come through.

Take time to enjoy your kids. Gratefulness comes into play here. Taking time to truly enjoy my kids has brought so much happiness to my life, and honestly, I didn't even know that I wasn't doing this before, it's only now that I've applied this practice to my everyday life and everyday parenting that I notice the difference. If you're thinking to yourself right now as you read this, I don't have time to sit and play with my kids, I'm swamped. I'm here to be that little tap on your shoulder that's saying, make time. Make time now because time is something you can't recreate or get back once it's gone. Move something around and spare fifteen to thirty minutes to play with kids. Helping with homework or teaching them how to pick up something doesn't count. I want you down in the floor with that fake spoon pretending to sip your fake tea. Don't think about what else you could be doing that I know needs done. You will have time later, funny thing about the universe and trusting the higher power, and I can say this with full confidence because this has and is happening in my life, when you do the right things like taking time to play with your kids, all the rest of the stuff falls into line, no I'm not saying your laundry magically washed and folds itself, but you have available time to do it without feeling overwhelmed that it's still a task on your schedule.

I'd like to conclude this chapter with one last topic: Getting embarrassed by things your kids say or do. It seems like this is something I see a lot of when I'm out in public or if we have friends over that bring their kids and while they are visiting their kids act up. Naturally kids do things that aren't always the most mannerly thing to do. We recently had some friends over that brought their little boy with them, he was in a particularly cranky mood, throwing tantrums and being whiney, he's two, so of course his behavior was true to his age and he probably was fighting sleep. His parents, our friends, became frustrated and left because they were embarrassed that he was acting that way. That's not the only time I've seen parents get embarrassed and act according to how being embarrassed by their child's behavior made them feel. It's important to allow your children to express their personalities and for them to be allowed to show their emotions without being scolded constantly because you're feeling embarrassed over their behavior. I know that this is a fine line. You can't let your kids misbehave terribly and run wild at some places. This isn't what I'm talking about, I'm talking about being at a store and your child getting upset and you letting it embarrass and upset you to the point that you become extremely frustrated and maybe even hateful toward your misbehaving kid. I've seen this all too often, especially recently, which is why I'm bringing it up. I've seen parent's pop their kids on the behind because they were trying to shop and there five-year-old was tired of looking at house décor, be real mammas, I know it's impossible to go into home-goods or pier one with a time limit; however, don't expect your little one to enjoy looking at flowers and throw pillows as much as you do. They are going to become restless.

This is where it's important for you to remind yourself that if you act out toward them while there having their meltdown, because they are embarrassing you in public and people are starring, you're going to embarrass them. It's going to be-little them and they are not going to understand what they are being popped on the bum for anyway. All they know is mom has been in this store for what seems like to them two whole days and they want to go play now, that's it. It's innocent and there is no alternative motive like, it's time for me to ruin moms shopping trip, behind it. Leave your buggy full of all your pretty, must-have items or walk whatever you can't live without to the front and ask someone to hold it, excuse yourself and take that baby to the car. Give him or her a break, then go back in or if you're on a time limit, come back later. There will be just as much there the next time as there was this time. The choice of walking away to tend to your child feels much better than scolding them in front of everyone for not acting like there 25 and understanding that they need to be quiet while you shop. Arrange your thoughts and actions to have a better reaction to these situations, not only for you, but for your little one.

Sometimes you can laugh at what may seem embarrassing. My sister-in-law recently came to my house for a visit and she brought my niece with her. While they were visiting, my oldest daughter had an eye appointment, so I asked my niece if she'd like to some with us and she did. Before we went to the doctor, I stopped at target for a couple things and allowed her and my daughter one item each. My nieces present was a squishy toy that sounded like toot's when you squeezed it. While we were in the doctor's office, she decided it would be a good time to try out her new favorite thing. She was sitting on my lap squeezing this toy and it truly sounded like huge toot's, it was also a little loud and the patient room door was open. About five minutes into this, really loud and in a purposefully deep voice and accent she says, "Aunt Katie, I don't know why, but I just can't quit farting."

Now, this could've gone one of two ways.

One. I could've gotten embarrassed. The doctors were standing right outside the door, so I know they heard the noises and probably thought it was me based on how loud this little squeeze toy was. I could've scolded her and told her not to do that because it wasn't appropriate and that it was embarrassing. Basically, I could've sucked all the fun from the situation.

Or, I could've done exactly what I did. Laugh hysterically with her. She's six. She thought it was the funniest thing ever. I could care less what those doctors thought. None of it mattered. All that mattered is my adorable niece was cuddled up on my lap, laughing hysterically while I got to share that moment with her. We laughed all day about that, it was really funny.

Choosing to not let embarrassment flood out everything else was the best decision. Let go of your reaction to what people may be thinking. If you're smiling and laughing and you feel happy and there's no harm coming to anyone, then why let anything or anyone ruin that moment for you? Enjoy it, we are human and every one of us has embarrassing stories we can tell, you're going to laugh about it later anyway, why not laugh about it now too.

TIP: Work on the things I've mentioned in this chapter, along with other things you may feel are prohibiting you in any area of parenting or your busy life. If it's patience, remember to meditate and quiet your chatter. If it's your limited time with your kids, remember to make the time and feel confident that the universe will work it out that you have time to finish up everything else later. Whatever the issue, just remember that these skills are not limited to helping heal only one problem. You can use them throughout your day on any block you may have.

Chapter Eleven
Perception: Enemy or Frenemy?

"What day is it?" asks Pooh.
"It's Today," says Christopher Robin.
"Oh, my favorite day," replies Pooh.
– *Christopher Robin and Pooh, The Disney Movie
'Christopher Robin'*

I read an article in the Huff Post that was titled 'I have a bachelor's degree and still work four jobs to make ends meet', it was about a girl who's life consisted around working, went to school to better herself and when she finally graduated with a bachelor's degree she thought, this is it, it's time for my finances, my job and my life to be better, but year after year she found herself stuck, in the same debt, the same dead end jobs, the same life she was so desperately trying to escape.

Do you find yourself saying this year will be better, this year will not contain the bills, dead ends, and nonproductive everything that has been a leech on my back? Do you feel like you're trying to escape?

You may not want to hear this, but the fact is, everything we have in our lives right now, house, car, money, family, clothes, knowledge, EVERYTHING, is there because we have made choices to bring it into our lives. We at some point made a choice based on whatever we felt at that time and attracted all we have and know to us. Then based on how we perceive these things we've place a judgment on each thing as good, bad, not necessary, necessary and so forth. Perception can be everything and nothing, depending on the hold you have to it.

Do you know why the girl from the huff post blog felt so enormously disappointed in her life? Her perception about all that she had, all she had accomplished and all that she didn't have was negative. All those negative perceptions had control of her focus. She, like so many others, had placed all her negative perceptions at the focal point in her life. Why is it that we allow a snowball effect to occur over these types of circumstances? Why do we focus and perceive any type of struggle or wishing something was different to be on the negative side? It's our perception – either our enemy or our frenemy.

I recently took a trip to visit my family in Florida. It was beautiful and a lust took hold on me that was unlike any I had experienced in terms of wanting so bad to live in a particular place. I mean, I just loved everything about it. It was warm, beautiful, near the prettiest beaches I had seen. I perceived it to be a paradise on earth. I spent most of my days that I was there looking at houses online and texting my mom to see if she and my dad would consider moving because I always prefer them near. I really took it to the next level. I pouted on the car ride home when my fantasy of moving seemed to slip through my fingers, I was negative and had a frustrating echo outpour all around me. Unfortunately for my family, they were stuck in the car with me and had to hold steady through this radiating negative vibe. I started finding myself wishing I hadn't even gone because then I wouldn't have known how nice it was and I wouldn't feel so upset over not getting to move there. This went on for a week! I allowed myself to fall into this negative, for me and everyone around me, emotion; perceiving the trip as a disappointment in that it hadn't worked out that we'd be moving. The whole thing rippled into a mess within.

I had to STOP. I halted my entire thought process when I realized that I was making everyone, including myself, miserable over something like this. What was I doing? Why was I allowing this to become such a negative focus? My perception of it. That's why. I started rethinking my trip. I thought about how I had become so consumed with my plan to move my family that I hadn't spent any time in the pool with my kids. I thought about how instead of texting my mom that I wish she could've been there to enjoy the beautiful weather and scenery, I sent about a hundred screenshots of houses I thought she'd like. I thought of the time I wasted and how I pulled everyone around me into my spiraling ripple. Wow did I feel crummy. *What the heck!* That was my first thought. Second thought was, *how do I fix this?* Then, I thought about perception. I perceived this trip as a negative thing because of what I had attached to it, negative thoughts and disappointment. Then it spiraled because I was feeding it all my focus. I stopped and retraced. I'm not going to lie, I felt very yucky knowing that

I had wasted precious time and what could've been beautiful moments with my family, it actually made me a little nauseous, but I couldn't go back.

All I could do is go forward and change my perception. In order to change perception, you must change your thoughts and the focus you have on them. It's just like I said in Chapter Seven, there is another way to look at the situation in front of you. I thought about my trip and I first allowed a feeling of gratitude to surface in the fact that I got an opportunity to go on a trip in the first place. Then, I thought about how I was fortunate to have my family together in such a beautiful place and that I was able to provide such a great trip for my children. I allowed this gratitude and joy to fill the previously filled disappointment hole. Next, I closed my eyes and took three deep breathes, I envisioned them to be healing breathes, forgiving myself for all the negative emotions I had allowed to seep in and out of me, that had an effect on me and others. I apologized for my behavior to my family and explained how I had let negative thoughts and emotions take over. After that, I started feeling much better, I shifted my perception of the trip from: It sucks that I'll never get to move there, to, I'm so grateful that I have an opportunity to visit such a beautiful place whenever I'd like. My perception changed my entire feeling for the better.

Perception and The Law of Attraction go hand in hand. Like attracts Like. If you perceive things negatively and then focus on that negative perception, you may be attracting negative emotions and situations to you. How you perceive things can have a huge impact on your everyday life. It can have a huge impact on your family's life. Your perception on things can create many emotions, good and not so good. It's very important that you harbor no judgments, no negative emotions, no negative thoughts that consume your focus. It's equally important to press STOP whenever you become aware of what's happening even if you're up to your neck in the water. It's never too late to change the course. Shift your perceptions on everything in your life to be more positive, shift them to bring about more positive emotions. Allow those perceptions to be the things you focus on. Approach each new situation with a positive perception, a glass half full kind of approach, anything else is a set up for something negative. It's never too late to change your perceptions. Growth is ever flowing on the spiritual journey; it's never too late for anything.

TIP:

- **Encounter**

  Next time you meet someone new, allow your perception to be open, allow peace and love for this fellow human being to be your focus. You don't have to hug them or anything, just allow your vibes to be good natured and free from any negative perceptions.

- **A New Situation**

  If you find yourself in a new situation, something you may not be accustom to, shift any perceptions you may be feeling bad about it, to more uplifting perceptions. Example: If you're feeling nervous to travel because it's something you've never done, try to make a shift to excitement for this new experience.

- **Perception of Another**

If you once had a partner that was unfaithful, and you now perceive all your partners to be unfaithful based on an experience you once had. Change your perception from judgment and fear to something more beneficial to your wellbeing. For example, allow yourself to understand that something was lacking and you've made a conscious decision to grow past the hurt and approach it with peace and knowledge that it couldn't have possibly been from the spirit and you are now able to recognize that and move past the block. This allows you to perceive your new partner openly, without a negative perception derived from the past that has no place in the now.

Chapter Twelve
The Beginning

Trust. Surrender. Utilize

Trust, that the spirit inside you, guides you. Trust equals Faith.

All that I am, all that I think I know, all that I know I know, all that I hope to become, I surrender to you, higher power. I surrender to peace, love, joy, courage, strength and faith. Show me true peace, show me true love, show me true joy, show me true strength, show me true faith, so that I can become them and apply them to every part of my life. I release my ideas of what I think these things are. I am hungry for spiritual knowledge. I humbly surrender.

Utilize your knowledge of spiritual truth. Put action behind your will to grow into a better human being with a purpose to help all human beings. You must put action behind spiritual truth for it to bring about change in you and in your life. Have trust in the awareness you seek, surrender your old self, habits and thoughts; utilize your newfound knowledge that has always been within you waiting for you to awaken.

That is your next step.

This is the beginning of your new life, the beginning of the new you.

Resources

This is a list of books, guided meditation links and video's that were of importance to me and still provide me with peace, comfort and solidness whenever I feel that I'm on shaky ground (having an off day). Just because you're on a journey to have a better life and become a better person doesn't mean you will no longer encounter moments that are out of alignment. What matters is how you handle those moments that you use your knowledge of spiritual awareness to stop old patterns from allowing a spiral effect, what matters is your new response when things go astray. I have read each book, watched each video and have meditated with each link I've listed; they are my favorite tools that I use thus far in my journey. I hope this book along with this list helps you. I wish only happiness for you and for your family and I truly appreciate you taking time to read this book and grow to become a more enlightened human being, after all, what helps us, helps our children and eventually all mankind. It's time to change the course for a brighter and more peaceful future.

All My Love! K.

- Eckhart Tolle. A New Earth (Book)
- Eckhart Tolle. Oneness with All Life (Book)
- Deepak Chopra – The Cosmic Mind and the Sub manifest Order of Being (Audiobook)
- Wayne W. Dyer. Your Erroneous Zones (Book)
- Roy Masters. Meaning and Happiness (Audiobook)
- Deepak Chopra. Living Without Limits (Book)
- Deepak Chopra. The Spontaneous Fulfillment of Desire (Book)
- ShefaliTsabary. The Conscious Parent (Book)
- ShefaliTsabary. The Awakened Family (Book)
- A Grateful Day with Brother David Steindl-Rast (YouTube Link: https://youtu.be/zSt7k_q_qRU)
- Guided Meditation for Anxiety and Stress, Beginning Meditation, Guided Imagery Visualization
  (YouTube Link: http://youtu.be/6vO1wPAmiMQ)
- The Secret. 2006 Documentary (Movie)
- Tony Robbins: I Am Not Your Guru – 2016 Documentary (Movie)